CERTIFIED SURGICAL TECHNOLOGIST

BY

ALFAJIRI PUBLISHERS

Copyright 2016. All rights reserved. No copy of this eBook, except for brief review, may be transmitted, reproduced, stored in a retrieval system, in any form or by any means- electronic, mechanical, photocopying, recording or otherwise- without the written permission of the publisher/author.

ALFAJIRI PUBLICATIONS
1510 WEST PAWNEE
WICHITA, KANSAS

TABLE OF CONTENTS

INTRODUCTION TO ANATOMY
SURGICAL TERMS
CARDIAC TERMINOLOGY
EQUIPMENT STERILIZATION
SURGICAL INSTRUMENTS
PREOPERATIVE CARE
INTRAOPERATIVE CARE
POSTOPERATIVE CARE
NEUROLOGY
MICROBIOLOGY
MICROBIOLOGY TERMS
PHARMACOLOGY
TESTS AND ANSWERS

INTRODUCTION TO ANATOMY

Skeletal System

When many people imagine anatomy, they think of a skeleton. Your skeletal system is made up of your bones. Bones give your body the structure and shape it needs to move. They also help to protect your soft internal organs. Your bones have a hard, powerful outer surface made of compact material that can withstand forces, and they have a jelly-like interior called bone marrow. There are 206 bones within an adult's body. In order to grow, bones need calcium, which can be found in milk.

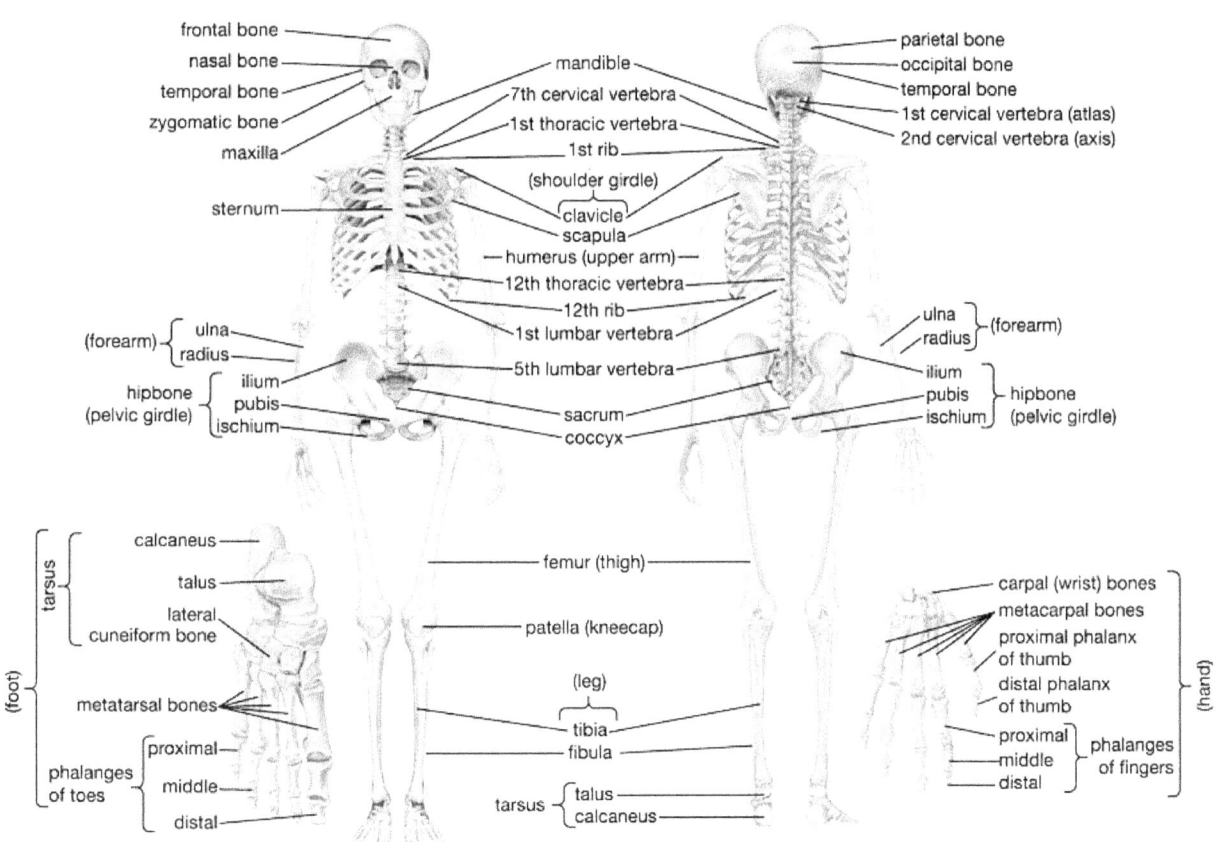

Muscular System

Muscles are made up of bundles of long, thin cells. Your body's motions come from muscles either contracting or relaxing. The muscles that move bones, such as in your arm, work in pairs together to produce movement. For example, as you raise your forearm, the muscle at the front of your upper arm, your bicep, contracts and forms a bulge. As you let your forearm back down, your tricep on the back of your upper arm will contract and your bicep will relax. In order to become stronger, people exercise. That exercise leads to tiny micro-tears in the fibers, which heal and become stronger.

Cardiovascular System

Your heart is a muscle, but it's also part of its own system: the cardiovascular system. Your heart's job is to pump blood, which will circulate throughout the body. Blood is pumped through arteries and capillaries and comes back to the heart through veins. Your heart is always working, so it's important to take proper care of it by exercising and eating well.

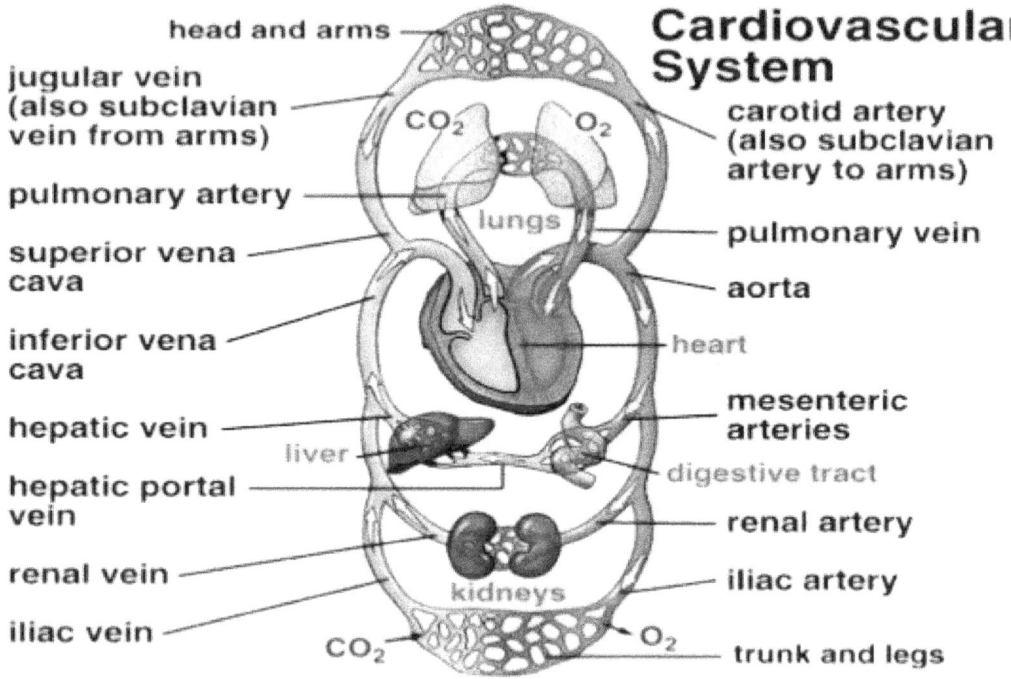

Digestive System

Your digestive system is very important and includes many different organs. Food travels from your mouth through your esophagus to your stomach, then into your intestines and your rectum. As it moves throughout the body, the food is digested. In other words, useable nutrients are absorbed into the bloodstream, and waste is disposed of as feces.

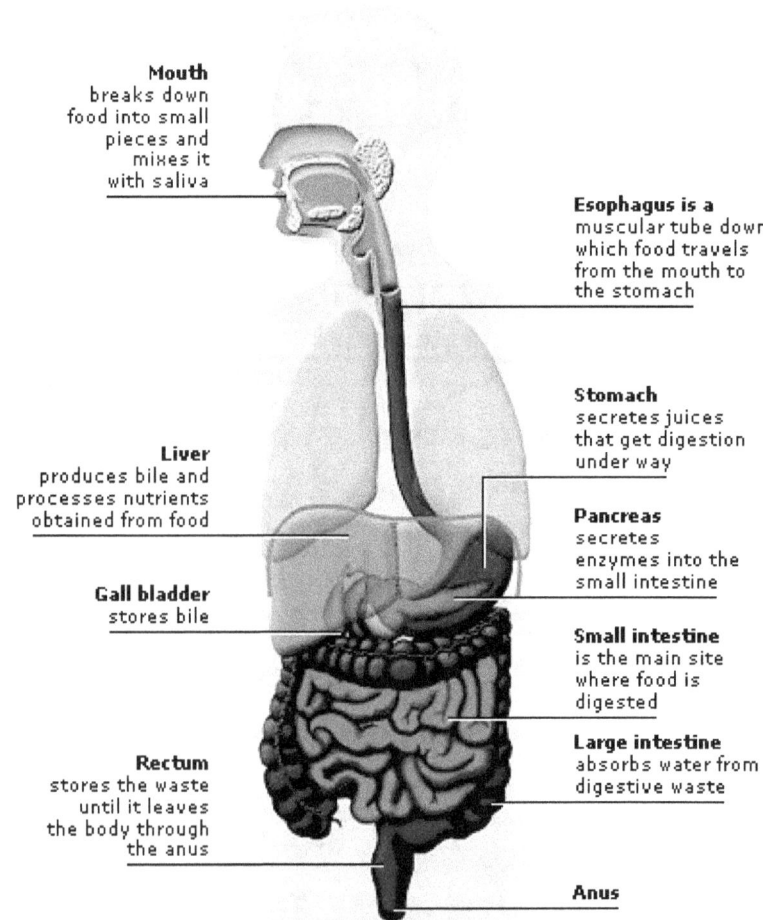

Respiratory System

Your body needs oxygen to function. The organs that are responsible for taking in and processing the air are part of the respiratory system. Those organs include the pharynx, larynx, trachea, bronchial tubes, and lungs. The lungs have a hard job to do: They absorb oxygen so that it can be sent to the heart and circulated throughout the body. The lungs can be harmed when breathing in bad chemicals, such as from cigarettes.

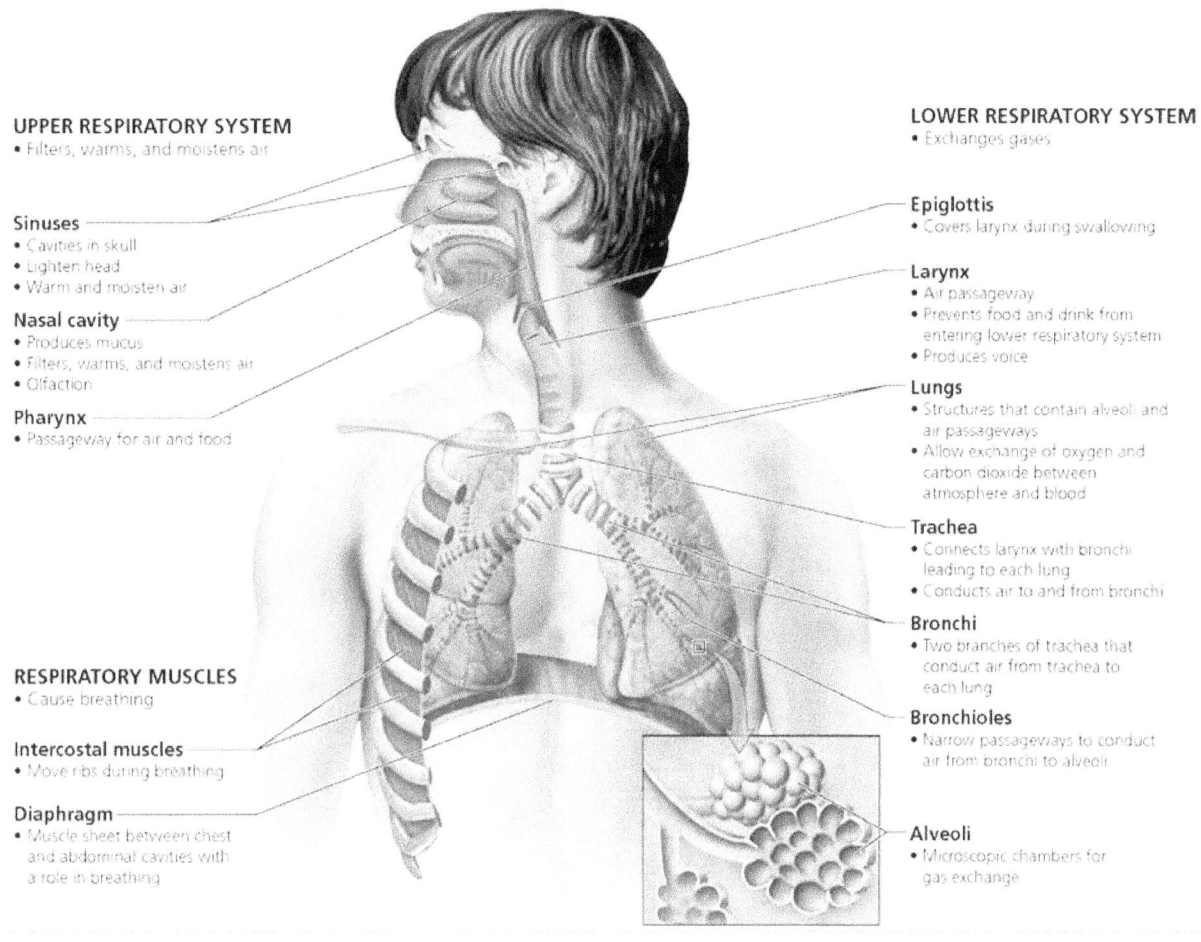

UPPER RESPIRATORY SYSTEM
- Filters, warms, and moistens air

Sinuses
- Cavities in skull
- Lighten head
- Warm and moisten air

Nasal cavity
- Produces mucus
- Filters, warms, and moistens air
- Olfaction

Pharynx
- Passageway for air and food

RESPIRATORY MUSCLES
- Cause breathing

Intercostal muscles
- Move ribs during breathing

Diaphragm
- Muscle sheet between chest and abdominal cavities with a role in breathing

LOWER RESPIRATORY SYSTEM
- Exchanges gases

Epiglottis
- Covers larynx during swallowing

Larynx
- Air passageway
- Prevents food and drink from entering lower respiratory system
- Produces voice

Lungs
- Structures that contain alveoli and air passageways
- Allow exchange of oxygen and carbon dioxide between atmosphere and blood

Trachea
- Connects larynx with bronchi leading to each lung
- Conducts air to and from bronchi

Bronchi
- Two branches of trachea that conduct air from trachea to each lung

Bronchioles
- Narrow passageways to conduct air from bronchi to alveoli

Alveoli
- Microscopic chambers for gas exchange

Nervous System

In addition to containing a vast network of arteries, veins, muscles, and bones, your body also contains a network of nerves, which touch almost every part of the body. The system can be broken up into two major systems: the central nervous system and the peripheral nervous system. The central nervous system contains the brain and spinal cord, which is the epicenter of nerve cells. Outside of that region is the peripheral nervous system where nerves often connect with other muscles and tissues. As human beings, we have fairly big brains, which allow us to read, think, and react to things.

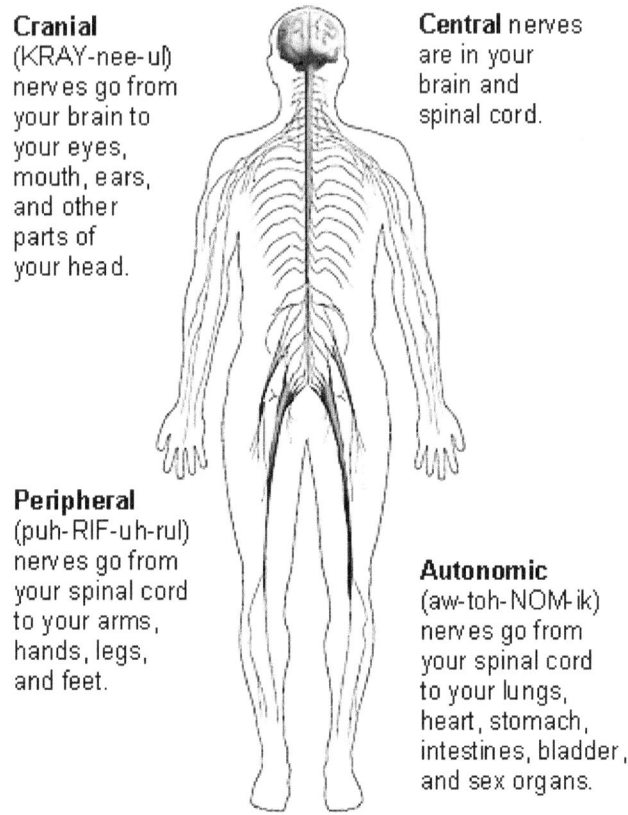

Cranial (KRAY-nee-ul) nerves go from your brain to your eyes, mouth, ears, and other parts of your head.

Central nerves are in your brain and spinal cord.

Peripheral (puh-RIF-uh-rul) nerves go from your spinal cord to your arms, hands, legs, and feet.

Autonomic (aw-toh-NOM-ik) nerves go from your spinal cord to your lungs, heart, stomach, intestines, bladder, and sex organs.

Excretory System

The excretory system is similar to the digestive system in that it's responsible for discharging wastes. The difference is that the excretory system gets rid of liquid waste. This system is responsible for keeping the chemical balance in the bloodstream. Related organs include the kidneys, skin, and bladder. Through urine and sweat, waste is excreted.

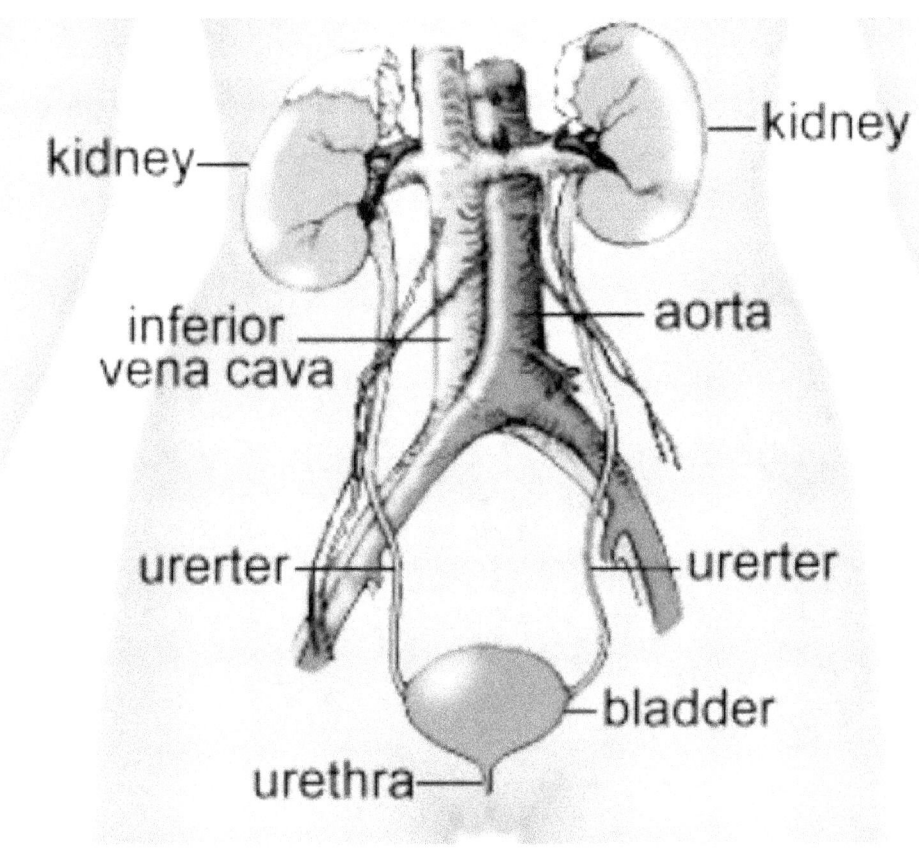

Humans Excretory System

Endocrine System

Growing up, you may hear a lot about hormones. Hormones are related to the endocrine system, which consists of a group of organs that communicate with chemical messages. There are quite a few organs in this system, all with their own unique chemical signature: the pineal gland, pituitary gland, hypothalamus, thymus, thyroid, adrenal glands, pancreas, and sex glands. This is one of the least-understood systems of the body, but we do know that these organs release chemicals into the bloodstream to let the rest of the body know what to do.

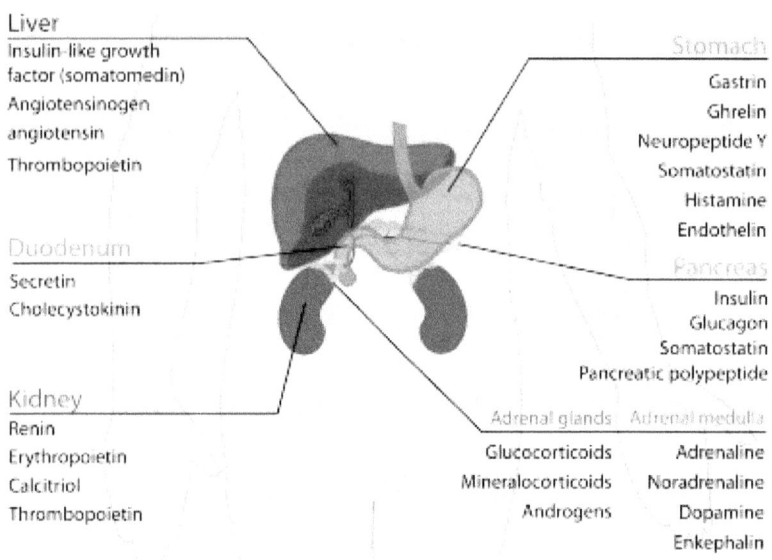

Liver
Insulin-like growth factor (somatomedin)
Angiotensinogen
angiotensin
Thrombopoietin

Duodenum
Secretin
Cholecystokinin

Kidney
Renin
Erythropoietin
Calcitriol
Thrombopoietin

Stomach
Gastrin
Ghrelin
Neuropeptide Y
Somatostatin
Histamine
Endothelin

Pancreas
Insulin
Glucagon
Somatostatin
Pancreatic polypeptide

Adrenal glands
Glucocorticoids
Mineralocorticoids
Androgens

Adrenal medulla
Adrenaline
Noradrenaline
Dopamine
Enkephalin

ANATOMY QUIZ

Questions

1) Which of the following terms describes the body's ability to maintain its normal state?

(A) Anabolism
(B) Catabolism
(C) Tolerance
(D) Homeostasis
(E) Metabolism

2) Which of the following best describes the human body's defense mechanism against environmental bacteria?

(A) Hair in the nose
(B) Mucous membranes
(C) Osteoblasts
(D) Saliva
(E) Tears

3) Which of the following best describes a nucleus cell?

(A) Lymphocyte
(B) Monocyte
(C) Erythrocyte
(D) Basophil
(E) Neutrophil

4) Which of the following is flexible connective tissue that is attached to bones at the joints?

(A) Adipose
(B) Cartilage
(C) Epithelial
(D) Muscle
(E) Nerve

5) Which of the following allows air to pass into the lungs?

(A) Aorta
(B) Esophagus
(C) Heart

(D) Pancreas
(E) Trachea

6) Which of the following is the body cavity that contains the pituitary gland?

(A) Abdominal
(B) Cranial
(C) Pleural
(D) Spinal
(E) Thoracic

7) Which of the following closes and seals off the lower airway during swallowing?

(A) Alveoli
(B) Epiglottis
(C) Larynx
(D) Uvula
(E) Vocal cords

8) Which of the following is located beneath the diaphragm in the left upper quadrant of the abdominal cavity?

(A) Appendix
(B) Kidney
(C) Liver
(D) Spleen
(E) Stomach

9) Which of the following anatomical regions of abdomen lies just distal to the sternum?

(A) Epigastric
(B) Hypochondriac
(C) Hypogastric
(D) Lumbar
(E) Umbilical

10) Which of the following cavities are separated by the diaphragm?

(A) Abdominal and pelvic
(B) Cranial and spinal
(C) Dorsal and ventral
(D) Pericardial and pleural
(E) Thoracic and abdominal

11) Which of the following terms describes the motion of bending the forearm toward the body?

(A) Abduction
(B) Eversion
(C) Flexion
(D) Pronation
(E) Supination

12) In which of the following positions does a patient lie face down?

(A) Dorsal
(B) Erect
(C) Lateral
(D) Prone
(E) Supine

13) If the foot is abducted, it is moved in which direction?

(A) Inward
(B) Outward
(C) Upward
(D) Downward

14) The anatomic location of the spinal canal is

(A) caudal
(B) dorsal
(C) frontal
(D) transverse
(E) ventral

15) Which of the following is a structural, fibrous protein found in the dermis?

(A) Collagen
(B) Heparin
(C) Lipocyte
(D) Melanin
(E) Sebum

16) A patient has a fracture in which the radius is bent but not displaced, and the skin is intact. This type of fracture is known as which of the following?

(A) Closed, greenstick
(B) Complex, comminuted
(C) Compound, transverse
(D) Open, spiral
(E) Simple, pathologic

17) Which of the following is the large bone found superior to the patella and inferior to the ischium?

(A) Calcaneus
(B) Femur
(C) Symphysis pubis
(D) Tibia
(E) Ulna

18) The physician directs the medical assistant to complete a request form for an X-ray study of the fibula. The procedure will be performed on which of the following structures?

(A) Heel
(B) Lower leg
(C) Toes
(D) Thigh
(E) Pelvis

19) Which of the following is a disorder characterized by uncontrollable episodes of falling asleep during the day?

(A) Dyslexia
(B) Epilepsy
(C) Hydrocephalus
(D) Narcolepsy
(E) Shingles

20) Which of the following is the point at which an impulse is transmitted from one neuron to another neuron?

(A) Dendrite
(B) Glial cell
(C) Nerve center
(D) Synapse
(E) Terminal plate

21) Which of the following controls body temperature, sleep, and appetite?

(A) Adrenal glands
(B) Hypothalamus
(C) Pancreas
(D) Thalamus
(E) Thyroid gland

22) Which of the following cranial nerves is related to the sense of smell?

(A) Abducens
(B) Hypoglossal
(C) Olfactory
(D) Trochlear
(E) Vagus

23) Which of the following is a substance that aids the transmission of nerve impulses to the muscles?

(A) Acetylcholine
(B) Cholecystokinin
(C) Deoxyribose
(D) Oxytocin
(E) Prolactin

24) Which of the following best describes the location where the carotid pulse can be found?

(A) In front of the ears and just above eye level
(B) In the antecubital space
(C) In the middle of the groin
(D) On the anterior side of the neck
(E) On the medial aspect of the wrist

25) A patient sustains severe blunt trauma to the left upper abdomen and requires surgery. Which one of the following organs is most likely to be involved?

(A) Appendix
(B) Gallbladder
(C) Pancreas
(D) Urinary bladder
(E) Spleen

26) Where is the sinoatrial node located?

(A) Between the left atrium and the left ventricle
(B) Between the right atrium and the right ventricle
(C) In the interventricular septum
(D) In the upper wall of the left ventricle
(E) In the upper wall of the right atrium

27) Blood flows from the right ventricle of the heart into which of the following structures?

(A) Inferior vena cava
(B) Left ventricle
(C) Pulmonary arteries
(D) Pulmonary veins
(E) Right atrium

28) Oxygenated blood is carried to the heart by which of the following structures?

(A) Aorta
(B) Carotid arteries
(C) Inferior vena cava
(D) Pulmonary veins
(E) Superior vena cava

29) The thoracic cage is a structural unit important for which of the following functions?

(A) Alimentation
(B) Menstruation
(C) Mentation
(D) Respiration
(E) Urination

30) Which of the following substances is found in greater quantity in exhaled air?

(A) Carbon dioxide
(B) Carbon monoxide
(C) Nitrogen
(D) Oxygen
(E) Ozone

31) Which of the following allows gas exchange in the lungs?

(A) Alveoli
(B) Bronchi
(C) Bronchioles

(D) Capillaries
(E) Pleurae

32) At which of the following locations does bile enter the digestive tract?

(A) Gastroesophageal sphincter
(B) Duodenum
(C) Ileocecum
(D) Jejunum
(E) Pyloric sphincter

33) Which of the following structures is part of the small intestine?

(A) Ascending colon
(B) Cecum
(C) Ileum
(D) Sigmoid colon
(E) Transverse colon

34) Which of the following conditions is characterized by incompetence of the esophageal sphincter?

(A) Crohn's disease
(B) Esophageal varices
(C) Gastroesophageal reflux disease
(D) Pyloric stenosis
(E) Stomatitis

35) Which of the following organs removes bilirubin from the blood, manufactures plasma proteins, and is involved with the production of prothrombin and fibrinogen?

(A) Gallbladder
(B) Kidney
(C) Liver
(D) Spleen
(E) Stomach

36) Which of the following is an accessory organ of the gastrointestinal system that is responsible for secreting insulin?

(A) Adrenal gland
(B) Gallbladder
(C) Liver

(D) Pancreas
(E) Spleen

37) Which of the following is the lymphoid organ that is a reservoir for red blood cells and filters organisms from the blood?

(A) Appendix
(B) Gallbladder
(C) Pancreas
(D) Spleen
(E) Thymus

38) Which of the following best describes the process whereby the stomach muscles contract to propel food through the digestive tract?

(A) Absorption
(B) Emulsion
(C) Peristalsis
(D) Regurgitation
(E) Secretion

39) Saliva contains an enzyme that acts upon which of the following nutrients?

(A) Starches
(B) Proteins
(C) Fats
(D) Minerals
(E) Vitamins

40) In men, specimens for gonococci cultures are most commonly obtained from which of the following structures?

(A) Anus
(B) Bladder
(C) Skin
(D) Testicle
(E) Urethra

41) Which of the following describes the cluster of blood capillaries found in each nephron in the kidney?

(A) Afferent arteriole
(B) Glomerulus

(C) Loop of Henley
(D) Renal pelvis
(E) Renal tubule

42) Which of the following conditions is characterized by the presence of kidney stones (renal calculi)?

(A) Glomerulonephritis
(B) Interstitial nephritis
(C) Nephrolithiasis
(D) Polycystic kidney
(E) Pyelonephritis

43) Which of the following best describes the structure that collects urine in the body?

(A) Bladder
(B) Kidney
(C) Ureter
(D) Urethra
(E) Urethral meatus

44) In men, which of the following structures is located at the neck of the bladder and surrounds the urethra?

(A) Epididymis
(B) Prostate
(C) Scrotum
(D) Seminal vesicle
(E) Vas deferens

45) Male hormones are produced by which of the following?

(A) Glans penis
(B) Prepuce
(C) Prostate
(D) Testes
(E) Vas deferens

46) which of the following are mucus-producing glands located on each side of the vaginal opening?

(A) Adrenal
(B) Bartholdi's

(C) Bulbourethral
(D) Corpus lutein
(E) Parotid

47) Fertilization of an ovum by a spermatozoon occurs in which of the following structures?

(A) Cervix
(B) Fallopian tube
(C) Ovary
(D) Uterus
(E) Vagina

48) Calcium, potassium, and sodium are classified as which of the following?

(A) Androgens
(B) Catecholamine's
(C) Electrolytes
(D) Estrogens
(E) Prostaglandins

49) Which of the following is the master gland of the endocrine system?

(A) Adrenal
(B) Pancreas
(C) Pineal
(D) Pituitary
(E) Thyroid

50) Patients with which of the following diseases are treated with injections of vitamin B-12?

(A) Bell's palsy
(B) Cohn's disease
(C) Diabetes mellitus
(D) Graves' disease
(E) Pernicious anemia

ANATOMY ANSWERS

1) D

2) B

3) C

4) B

5) E

6) B

7) B

8) C

9) A

10) E

11) C

12) D

13) B

14) B

15) A

16) A

17) B

18) B

19) D

20) D

21) B

22) C

23) A

24) D

25) E

26) E

27) C

28) D

29) D

30) A

31) A

32) B

33) C

34) C

35) C

36) D

37) D

38) C

39) A

40) E

41) B

42) C

43) A

44) B

45) D

46) B

47) B

48) C

49) D

50) E

SURGICAL TERMS

Surgical Terms

A list of common surgical terms, including the meaning and origin of prefixes and suffixes.

PREFIXES

A-/An-	not, without, less, absent: also, in a particular place or condition (Old English, from an, an alternative for on)
Ab-	Away from, off (Indo-European 'off, away')
Ad-	To, toward (Latin ad, 'toward, near')
Aer-	Air
Amb-	Both, on both sides
Amph-	On both sides
Angio-	To do with arteries
Ante-	Before
Anti-	Against, opposite (Greek anti, 'opposite, against')
Apo-	From, opposed
Auto-	Self
Bi-	Twice, double
Brachy-	Short (Greek brakhus 'short')
Brady-	Slow
Cardio-	The heart
Cata-	Down, back, apart (Greek kata)
Cephal-	The head
Chole-	To do with bile
Chromo-	Colour
Circum-	Around
Colo-	To do with the colon
Con-	Together
Cyan-	Blue (Greek kuanos, 'dark blue')
Contra-	Against
Cyst-	Bag, bladder
Cyto-	Cell
Dacry-	Tears
Dactyl-	Finger or toe (Greek daktulos)
De-	From, not
Deci-	Tenth
Demi-	Half
Dent-	Teeth

Derma-	Skin
Di-	Two, twice, double
Dia-	Through, across (Greek dia)
Diplo-	Double
Dis-	Apart, absence of
Docho-	Relating to a duct
Dys-	Bad or abnormal (Greek dus-)
Ect-, Ecto-	External, outside (Greek ektos 'out')
Eu-	Normal
Endo-	In, within, inside (Greek endo)
Entero-	Small intestine (Greek enteron. 'in, inside')
Epi-	On, over, above (Greek epi, 'upon')
Ex, exo-	Out
Extra-	Beyond or outside (Latin extra, 'outside, beyond')
Fore-	Before, in front of
Galacto-	Milk
Gastro-	The stomach
Genic-	Producing or related to genes (Greek genos, 'offspring, race')
Glosso-	The tongue
Haem-	Blood (Greek haima)
Hemi-	Half, partial (Greek hemi-)
Hepato-	Liver
Hetero-	Other, dissimilar
Holo-	All
Homo-	Same, similar
Hydro-	Water or liquid (Greek hudor)
Hyper-	Above or excessive (Greek huper)
Hypo-	Under or low (Greek hupo)
Idio-	Private or individual (Greek idios, 'one's own, private')
Ileo-	The ileum
Infra-	Beneath
Inter-	Between, among (Latin inter, 'between, among')
Intra-	Within or inside (Latin intra)
Intro-	Into or inward (Latin intro)
Iso-	Equal
Juxtra-	Near
Kerato-	Horn-like tissue, cornea (Greek keras, 'horn')
Kinese-	Movement

Lact-	Milk
Laparo-	Abdomen, loin
Laryngo-	Larynx
Latero-	Side
Lepto-	Thin, light, frail
Leuko-	White
Litho-	Stone or callculus (Greek lithos, 'stone')
Macro-	Large
Mal-	Bad
Medi-	Middle
Mega-	Large
Melano-	Black
Meno-	Menopause
Meso-	Middle, intermediate (Greek mesos)
Meta-	Later, behind (Greek meta, 'beside, after')
Micro-	Small
Mio-	Less, smaller
Mono-	Single
Multi-	Many
Myco-	Fungus, fungi (Greek mukes. 'slimy')
Myo-	Muscle
Myelo-	Marrow
Myxo-	Mucus
Neo-	New, recent (Greek neos)
Nephro-	Kidney
Neuro-	Nerves
Non-	No
Ob-	Against
Oculo-	Eye
Odont-	Tooth
Oligo-	Few
Omo-	Shoulder
Oo-	Ovum, egg (Greek oion)
Opisth-	Backward
Orchid-	Testicle
Ortho-	Correct; straight (Greek orthos, 'straight, right')
Os-	Mouth, bone
Osteo-	Bone (Greek osteon)

Oxy-	Sharp
Pachy-	Thick
Pan-	All (Greek 'all')
Para-	Beside, faulty (Greek para)
Path-	Disease
Per-	Going through a structure
Peri-	Around (Greek peri)
Pleo-	More
Pneu-, Pneumo-	Lungs, breathing
Pod-	Foot
Poikilo-	Iregular, varied
Poly-	More than one (Greek polus, 'much')
Post-	After
Pre-	Before
Pro-	Before
Procto-	Anus, rectum (Greek proktos)
Proto-	First
Pseudo-	False, spurious (Greek pseud 'to lie')
Psych-	Mind
Py-	Pus
Pyelo-	Relating to the pelvis of the kidney
Re-	Again
Retro-	Backward
Rhino-	Nose, nasal (Greek rhis, 'nose')
Sacro-	Sacrum
Salpingo-	Fallopian tube
Sarco-	Flesh
Sclero-	Hard
Scoto-	Darkness
Somato-	Relating to the body
Steato-	Fat (Greek steat)
Stetho-	Chest
Sub-	Under, below, beneath (Latin sub, 'under')
Supra-	Over, on top of (Latin supra, 'above, beyond')
Syn-	With, together
Tachy-	Accelerated, rapid (Greek takhus, 'swift')
Tampon-	To plug (French tampon)

Thermo-	Heat
Thyro-	Thyroid
Trans-	Going across a structure (Latin trans, 'across, over, through')
Tropho-	Nourishment, nutrition
Uni-	One, single (Latin unus)
Uro-	Urine
Vaso-	A vessel
Verm-	Worm-like
Xanth-	Yellow

SUFFIXES

-aceous	Resembling (Latin, 'related to')
-ade	An action (Latin –ata)
-aemia	Blood (Greek haima, 'blood')
-aesthesia, -esthesia	Sensation
-agogue	Substance promoting a flow of something (Greek agogos, 'a drawing off')
-algia	Pain (Greek algos, 'pain')
-cardial	Relating to the heart (Greek kardia, 'heart')
-cele	Tumor, cyst, hernia
-cephalic	Head (Greek kephale, 'head')
-cide	Causing death
-coel(e)	A cavity (Greek koilos, 'hollow') e.g. hydrocoele
-cyst	A fluid filled sac
-cyte	Cell e.g. phagocyte
-creas	Flesh (Greek kreas, 'flesh') e.g. pancreas
-dynia	Pain
-ectasia	Dilatation of ducts
-ectomy	Surgical excision of a part of the body (Latin -ectomia, 'cutting out') e.g. tonsillectomy – excision of the tonsils
-fuge	To drive away
-genic	The capacity to produce (Greek -genus, 'born')
-gogue	To make flow
-gram	An imaging technique using contrast medium
-itis	Inflammation (Greek) e.g. appendicitis (inflammation of the appendix)
-lasis	Condition, pathological state
-lysis	Set free, disintegrate

-megaly	Anormal enlargement (Greek megal-) e.g. splenomegaly
-morphic	Something that has a particular form, shape, or structure (Greek morphe) e.g. pleomorphic
-nexal	From 'nexus' indicating a connection or link e.g. adnexal
-oid	Shape, resemblance
-oma	A tumour (Latin) e.g. hepatoma – a tumour of the liver
-osis	Abnormal condition, process (Greek)
-oscopy	Inspection of a cavity
-ostomy	A connection between two hollow organs e.g. cholecystoduodenostomy – an anastomosis between the gall bladder and the duodenum
-ostosis	Formation of bone (Greek osteon, 'bone')
-otomy	To cut into a part of the body (Latin -tomia, 'cutting') e.g. laparotomy – an incision into the peritoneum
-penia	Lack
-phagia	Eating (Greek phagein 'to eat')
-pathy	Disorder or disease (Greek pathos)
-plasia	Growth or formation (Greek plassein, 'to form, mould')
-plasty	Surgical revision e.g. pyloroplasty (Greek plastos, 'refashion')
-plegia	Paralysis
-pnoea	Breath, respiration
-poiesis	Production
-rhage	Flow
-rhaphy	Suturing
-rrhoea	Flow, discharge (Greek rhein, 'to flow')
-sclerosis	Dryness, hardness
-scopy	To see
-stomosis	To create an outlet
-systole	Contraction of the heart (Greek sustole 'to contract')
-tomy	Cutting
-trophic	Nourishment
-tropic	Having an affinity for, turning towards
-uretic	To do with urine

TERMS

Abscess	A localised collection of pus (Latin abscessus, 'to go away' - referring to bodily humours going away in the pus)
Adenoma	A benign epithelial tumour of glandular origin
Aneurysm	Dilatation of an artery (Greek aneurusma, 'dilation,

	swelling')
Antegrade	Going in the direction of flow, e.g. antegrade pyelogram
Arrhythmia	Disturbance or irregularity of the heartbeat
Axillary	Of, relating to, or located near the axilla (armpit)
Ballotment	To toss about (French)
Bifurcation	To divide into two parts or branches
Biliary	Of or relating to bile, the bile ducts, or the gallbladder
Cannulation	The insertion of a cannula or tube into a hollow body organ
Capillary	A tube of small internal diameter
Cirrhosis	Chronic degenerative disease of the liver
Claudication	Claudius I (10BC – 54AD), Emperor of Rome had a limp, possibly due to polio. Hence the Latin term claudus for 'lame'.
Colitis	Inflammation of the colon
Concomitant	Occurring or existing concurrently
Cutaneous	Relating to or existing on or affecting the skin
Diverticulum	Plural diverticula (hence, use of the term 'diverticulae' is erroneous)
Dysplasia	Abnormal development or growth of tissues, organs, or cells
Embolus	A blood clot that becomes lodged in a blood vessel and obstructs it (Greek embolos, 'peg, stopper, wedge')
Empyema	A collection of pus in a body cavity
Endarterectomy	Surgical removal of the inner lining of an artery that is clogged with atherosclerosis
En bloc	On mass; all together
Fistula	A pipe or tube (Latin), plural fistulae. An abnormal communication between two hollow viscera, or one hollow viscera and the skin. It is conventional to name the diseased viscus first i.e. colovesical fistula due to diverticula disease; whereas, vesicocolic fistula from a bladder cancer.
Fundoplication	A surgical procedure involving making tucks in the fundus of the stomach around the lower end of the oesophagus
Ganglioma	A tumour of a ganglion
Gangrene	Death of tissue with putrefaction, sometimes referred to as 'wet' gangrene (Greek gaggraina, 'death of tissue'). C.f. necrosis, mummification
Haematoma	A swelling containing blood

Haemorrhage	Heavy bleeding from ruptured blood vessels
Haemorrhoid	Pain caused by venous swelling at or inside the anal sphincter
Hepatic	Of, relating to, or resembling the liver; acting on or occurring in the liver
Hernia	The abnormal protrusion of the contents of a cavity beyond the normal confines of that cavity
Hydatid	Cyst filled with liquid; forms as a result of infestation by tapeworm larvae
Ileus	Intestinal obstruction
Infarction	Infarct: localized necrosis resulting from obstruction of the blood supply
Inguinal	Of, relating to, or located in the groin
Intussusception	The enfolding of one segment of the intestine within another
Ischaemia	An inadequate supply of blood to a part of the body caused by blockage of an artery
Keloid	An area of raised pink or red fibrous scar tissue at the edges of a wound or incision (Greek khele, 'crab claw')
Laparoscopy	Laparotomy performed with a laparoscope that makes a small incision to examine the abdominal cavity
Lymphoma	Any of various usually malignant tumours that arise in the lymph nodes or in other lymphoid tissue
Maxillary	Of or relating to a jaw or jawbone, especially the upper one
Mesenteric	Of or relating to or located in a mesentery
Mesothelioma	A form of carcinoma of the mesothelium lining lungs or abdomen or heart; usually associated with exposure to asbestos dust
Metastasis	The spreading of a disease (especially cancer) to another part of the body
Mummification	Death of tissue with desiccation rather than putrefaction, sometimes referred to as 'dry' gangrene. (French momifier, 'to dry out and shrivel')
Necrosis	Death of tissue with structural evidence of such death
Nephrectomy	Surgical removal of a kidney
Occlusion	Closure or blockage (as of a blood vessel)
Omental	Pertaining to the omentum (a fold of peritoneum supporting the viscera)

Ossification	The developmental process of bone formation
Paediatric	Of or relating to the medical care of children
Perfusion	Pumping a liquid into an organ or tissue (especially by way of blood vessels)
Peritoneal	Of or relating to or affecting the peritoneum
Popliteal	Of or relating to the area behind the knee joint
Psoas	Either of two muscles of the abdomen and pelvis that flex the trunk and rotate the thigh
Retrograde	Going a reverse direction against flow e.g. endoscopic retrograde cholangiopancreatogram (ERCP)
Sebaceous	Greasy
Sepsis	The presence of pus-forming bacteria or their toxins in the blood or tissues
Sigmoid	Curved in two directions (like the letter S)
Sinus	A blind tract lined with granulation tissue hollow or gulf (Latin, 'curve, fold, hollow')
Slough	A piece of dead soft tissue or water (Old English sloh, a hole or low area in the ground filled with mud)
Splenic	Of or relating to the spleen
Squamous	Covered with or formed of scales; scaly
Stent	An artificial tube inserted into a tubular organ to keep it open
Stoma	Surgical opening: an artificial opening made in an organ, especially an opening in the colon (colostomy) or ileum (ileostomy) made via the abdomen. (Greek, 'mouth'). Plural stomata
Subacute	Used to describe a medical condition that develops less rapidly and with less severity than an acute condition
Suture	The fine thread or other material used surgically to close a wound or join tissues; an immovable joint (especially between the bones of the skull)
Thrombus	A blood clot that forms in a blood vessel and remains at the site of formation (Greek thrombos, 'clot')
Tomography	Obtaining pictures of the interior of the body
Tonsillar	Of or pertaining to the tonsils
Ulcer	A non-traumatic discontinuity of an epithelial surface (Latin ulcer, 'a sore')
Varicose veins	Dilated, lengthened, and tortuous veins

Ventricular Of or relating to a ventricle (of the heart or brain)

CARDIAC TERMINOLOGY

Abdomen - The area of the body between the bottom of the ribs and the top of the thighs.

Abdominal aorta - The portion of the aorta in the abdomen.

Ablation - Elimination or removal.

ACE (angiotensin-converting enzyme) inhibitor - A medicine that lowers blood pressure by interfering with the breakdown of a protein-like substance involved in blood pressure regulation.

Acetylcholine - A type of chemical (called a neurotransmitter) that transmits messages among nerve cells and muscle cells.

Acquired heart disease - Heart disease that arises after birth, usually from infection or through the build-up of fatty deposits in the arteries that feed the heart muscle.

Alveoli - Air sacs in the lungs where oxygen and carbon dioxide are exchanged.

Amiodarone - A kind of medicine (called an antiarrhythmic) used to treat irregular heart rhythms such as atrial fibrillation and ventricular tachycardia. It works by regulating nerve impulses in your heart. Amiodarone is mainly given to patients who have not responded to other antiarrhythmic medicines.

Aneurysm - A sac-like protrusion from a blood vessel or the heart, resulting from a weakening of the vessel wall or heart muscle.

Angina or angina pectoris - Chest pain that occurs when diseased blood vessels restrict blood flow to the heart.

Angiography - An x-ray technique in which dye is injected into the chambers of your heart or the arteries that lead to your heart (the coronary arteries). The test lets doctors measure the blood flow and blood pressure in the heart chambers and see if the coronary arteries are blocked.

Angioplasty - A nonsurgical technique for treating diseased arteries by temporarily inflating a tiny balloon inside an artery.

Angiotensin II receptor blocker - A medicine that lowers blood pressure by blocking the action of angiotensin II, a chemical in the body that causes the blood vessels to tighten (constrict).

Annulus - The ring around a heart valve where the valve leaflet merges with the heart muscle.

Antiarrhythmics - Medicines used to treat patients who have irregular heart rhythms.

Anticoagulant - Any medicine that keeps blood from clotting; a blood thinner.

Antihypertensive - Any medicine or other therapy that lowers blood pressure.

Antiplatelet therapy - Medicines that stop blood cells (called platelets) from sticking together and forming a blood clot.

Aorta - The largest artery in the body and the main vessel to supply blood from the heart.

Aortic valve - The valve that regulates blood flow from the heart into the aorta.

Aphasia - The inability to speak, write, or understand spoken or written language because of brain injury or disease.

Arrhythmia (or dysrhythmia) - An abnormal heartbeat.

Arrhythmogenic right ventricular dysplasia (ARVD) - ARVD is a type of cardiomyopathy with no known cause. It appears to be a genetic condition (passed down through a family's genes). ARVD causes ventricular arrhythmias.

Arteriography - A test that is combined with cardiac catheterization to visualize an artery or the arterial system after injection of a contrast dye.

Arterioles - Small, muscular branches of arteries. When they contract, they raise resistance to blood flow, and blood pressure in the arteries increases.

Artery - A vessel that carries oxygen-rich blood to the body.

Arteritis - Inflammation of the arteries.

Arteriosclerosis - A disease process, commonly called "hardening of the arteries", which includes a variety of conditions that cause artery walls to thicken and lose elasticity.

Artificial heart - A manmade heart. Also called a total artificial heart (TAH).

Ascending aorta - The first portion of the aorta, emerging from the heart's left ventricle.

Aspirin - Acetylsalicylic acid; a medicine used to relieve pain, reduce inflammation, and prevent blood clots.

Atherectomy - A nonsurgical technique for treating diseased arteries with a rotating device that cuts or shaves away material that is blocking or narrowing an artery.

Atherosclerosis - A disease process that leads to the buildup of a waxy substance, called plaque, inside blood vessels.

Atrium (right and left) - The two upper or holding chambers of the heart (together referred to as atria).

Atrial flutter - A type of arrhythmia in which the upper chambers of the heart (the atria) beat very fast, causing the walls of the lower chambers (the ventricles) to beat inefficiently as well.

Atrial septal defect - See septal defect.

Atrial tachycardia - A type of arrhythmia that begins in the heart's upper chambers (the atria) and causes a very fast heart rate of 160 to 200 beats a minute. A resting heart rate is normally 60 to 100 beats a minute.

Atrioventricular block - An interruption or disturbance of the electrical signal between the heart's upper two chambers (the atria) and lower two chambers (the ventricles).

Atrioventricular (AV) node - A group of cells in the heart located between the upper two chambers (the atria) and the lower two chambers (the ventricles) that regulates the electrical current that passes through it to the ventricles.

Atrium - Either one of the heart's two upper chambers.

Autologous - Relating to self. For example, autologous stem cells are those taken from the patient's own body.

Autoregulation - When blood flow to an organ stays the same although pressure in the artery that delivers blood to that organ may have changed.

Bacteria - Germs that can lead to disease.

Bacterial endocarditis - A bacterial infection of the lining of the heart's chambers (called the endocardium) or of the heart's valves.

Balloon catheter - A long tube-like device with a small balloon on the end that can be threaded through an artery. Used in angioplasty or valvuloplasty.

Balloon valvuloplasty - A procedure to repair a heart valve. A balloon-tipped catheter is threaded through an artery and into the heart. The balloon is inflated to open and separate any narrowed or stiffened flaps (called leaflets) of a valve.

Beta-blocker - An antihypertensive medicine that limits the activity of epinephrine, a hormone that increases blood pressure.

Biopsy - The process by which a small sample of tissue is taken for examination.

Blalock-Taussig procedure - A shunt between the subclavian and pulmonary arteries used to increase the supply of oxygen-rich blood in "blue babies" (see below).

Blood clot - A jelly-like mass of blood tissue formed by clotting factors in the blood. Clots stop the flow of blood from an injury. Clots can also form inside an artery when the artery's walls are damaged by atherosclerotic buildup, possibly causing a heart attack or stroke.

Blood pressure - The force or pressure exerted by the heart in pumping blood; the pressure of blood in the arteries.

Blue babies - Babies who have a blue tinge to their skin (cyanosis) resulting from insufficient oxygen in the arterial blood. This condition often indicates a heart defect.

Body mass index (BMI) - A number that indicates an increased risk of cardiovascular disease from a person being overweight. BMI is calculated using a formula of weight in kilograms divided by height in meters squared (BMI =W [kg]/H [m^2]). Click here for a BMI calculator.

Bradycardia - Abnormally slow heartbeat.

Bridge to transplant - Use of mechanical circulatory support to keep heart failure patients alive until a donor heart becomes available.

Bruit - A sound made in the blood vessels resulting from turbulence, perhaps because of a buildup of plaque or damage to the vessels.

Bundle branch block - A condition in which parts of the heart's conduction system are defective and unable to conduct the electrical signal normally, causing an irregular heart rhythm (arrhythmia).

Bypass - Surgery that can improve blood flow to the heart (or other organs and tissues) by providing a new route, or "bypass" around a section of clogged or diseased artery.

Calcium channel blocker (or calcium blocker) - A medicine that lowers blood pressure by regulating calcium-related electrical activity in the heart.

Capillaries - Microscopically small blood vessels between arteries and veins that distribute oxygen-rich blood to the body's tissues.

Cardiac - Pertaining to the heart.

Cardiac amyloidosis - A disorder caused by deposits of an abnormal protein (amyloid) in the heart tissue, which make it hard for the heart to work properly. Also called "stiff heart syndrome."

Cardiac arrest - The stopping of the heartbeat, usually because of interference with the electrical signal (often associated with coronary heart disease).

Cardiac cachexia - A term for the muscle and weight loss caused by severe heart disease. It is often related to the depressed cardiac output associated with end-stage heart failure, but it can also occur with severe coronary artery disease.

Cardiac catheterization - A procedure that involves inserting a fine, hollow tube (catheter) into an artery, usually in the groin area, and passing the tube into the heart. Often used along with angiography and other procedures, cardiac catheterization has become a primary tool for visualizing the heart and blood vessels and diagnosing and treating heart disease.

Cardiac enzymes - Complex substances capable of speeding up certain biochemical processes in the heart muscle. Abnormal levels of these enzymes signal heart attack.

Cardiac output - The amount of blood the heart pumps through the circulatory system in one minute.

Cardiologist - A doctor who specializes in the study of the heart and its function in health and disease.

Cardiology - The study of the heart and its function in health and disease.

Cardiomegaly - An enlarged heart. It is usually a sign of an underlying problem, such as high blood pressure, heart valve problems, or cardiomyopathy.

Cardiomyopathy - A disease of the heart muscle that leads to generalized deterioration of the muscle and its pumping ability.

Cardiopulmonary bypass - The process by which a machine is used to do the work of the heart and lungs so the heart can be stopped during surgery.

Cardiopulmonary resuscitation (CPR) - An emergency measure that can maintain a person's breathing and heartbeat. The person who performs CPR actually helps the patient's circulatory system by breathing into the patient's mouth to give them oxygen and by giving chest compressions to circulate the patient's blood. Hands-only CPR involves only chest compressions.

Cardiovascular (CV) - Pertaining to the heart and blood vessels that make up the circulatory system.

Cardiovascular Disease (CVD) - A general term referring to conditions affecting the heart (cardio) and blood vessels (vascular system). May also simply be called heart disease. Examples include coronary artery disease, valve disease, arrhythmia, peripheral vascular disease, congenital heart defects, hypertension, and cardiomyopathy. Refer to specific conditions for detailed explanations.

Cardioversion - A technique of applying an electrical shock to the chest to convert an abnormal heartbeat to a normal rhythm.

Carotid artery - A major artery (right and left) in the neck supplying blood to the brain.

Cerebral embolism - A blood clot formed in one part of the body and then carried by the bloodstream to the brain, where it blocks an artery.

Cerebral hemorrhage - Bleeding within the brain resulting from a ruptured blood vessel, aneurysm, or head injury.

Cerebral thrombosis - Formation of a blood clot in an artery that supplies part of the brain.

Cerebrovascular - Pertaining to the blood vessels of the brain.

Cerebrovascular accident - Also called cerebral vascular accident, apoplexy, or stroke. Blood supply to some part of the brain is slowed or stopped, resulting in injury to brain tissue.

Cerebrovascular occlusion - The blocking or closing of a blood vessel in the brain.

Cholesterol - An oily substance that occurs naturally in the body, in animal fats and in dairy products, and that is transported in the blood. Limited amounts are essential for the normal development of cell membranes. Excess amounts can lead to coronary artery disease.

Cineangiography - The technique of using moving pictures to show how a special dye passes through blood vessels, allowing doctors to diagnose diseases of the heart and blood vessels.

Circulatory system - Pertaining to circulation of blood through the heart and blood vessels.

Claudication - A tiredness or pain in the arms and legs caused by an inadequate supply of oxygen to the muscles, usually due to narrowed arteries or peripheral arterial disease (PAD).

Collateral circulation - Blood flow through small, nearby vessels in response to blockage of a main blood vessel.

Commissurotomy - A procedure used to widen the opening of a heart valve that has been narrowed by scar tissue.

Computed tomography (CT or CAT scan) - An x-ray technique that uses a computer to create cross-sectional images of the body.

Conduction system - Special muscle fibers that conduct electrical impulses throughout the heart muscle.

Congenital - Refers to conditions existing at birth.

Congenital heart defects - Malformation of the heart or of its major blood vessels present at birth.

Congestive heart failure - A condition in which the heart cannot pump all the blood returning to it, leading to a backup of blood in the vessels and an accumulation of fluid in the body's tissues, including the lungs.

Coronary arteries - Two arteries arising from the aorta that arch down over the top of the heart and divide into branches. They provide blood to the heart muscle.

Coronary artery anomaly (CAA) - A congenital defect in one or more of the coronary arteries of the heart.

Coronary artery bypass (CAB) - Surgical rerouting of blood around a diseased vessel that supplies blood to the heart. Done by grafting either a piece of vein from the leg or a piece of the artery from under the breastbone.

Coronary artery disease (CAD) - A narrowing of the arteries that supply blood to the heart. The condition results from a buildup of plaque and greatly increases the risk of a heart attack.

Coronary heart disease - Disease of the heart caused by a buildup of atherosclerotic plaque in the coronary arteries that can lead to angina pectoris or heart attack.

Coronary occlusion - An obstruction of one of the coronary arteries that hinders blood flow to the heart muscle.

Coronary thrombosis - Formation of a clot in one of the arteries carrying blood to the heart muscle. Also called coronary occlusion.

Cryoablation - The removal of tissue using an instrument called a cold probe.

Cyanosis - Blueness of the skin caused by a lack of oxygen in the blood.

Cyanotic heart disease - A birth defect of the heart that causes oxygen-poor (blue) blood to circulate to the body without first passing through the lungs.

Death rate (age-adjusted) - A death rate that has been standardized for age so different populations can be compared or the same population can be compared over time.

Deep vein thrombosis - A blood clot in a deep vein in the calf (DVT).

Defibrillator - A device that helps restore a normal heart rhythm by delivering an electric shock.

Diabetes (diabetes mellitus) - A disease in which the body doesn't produce or properly use insulin. Insulin is needed to convert sugar and starch into the energy used in daily life.

Diastolic blood pressure - The lowest blood pressure measured in the arteries. It occurs when the heart muscle is relaxed between beats.

Digitalis - A medicine made from the leaves of the foxglove plant. Digitalis is used to treat congestive heart failure (CHF) and heart rhythm problems (arrhythmias).

Dissecting aneurysm - A condition in which the layers of an artery separate or are torn, causing blood to flow between the layers. Dissecting aneurysms usually happen in the aorta, the large vessel that carries blood from the heart to other parts of the body and can cause sudden death.

Diuretic - A drug that lowers blood pressure by causing fluid loss. Diuretics promote urine production.

Doppler ultrasound - A technology that uses sound waves to assess blood flow within the heart and blood vessels and to identify leaking valves.

Dysarthria - A speech disorder resulting from muscular problems caused by damage to the brain or nervous system.

Dyspnea - Shortness of breath.

Echocardiography - A method of studying the heart's structure and function by analyzing sound waves bounced off the heart and recorded by an electronic sensor placed on the chest. A computer processes the information to produce a one-, two- or three-dimensional moving picture that shows how the heart and heart valves are functioning.

Edema - Swelling caused by fluid accumulation in body tissues.

Ejection fraction - A measurement of the rate at which blood is pumped out of a filled ventricle. The normal rate is 50% or more.

Electrocardiogram (ECG or EKG) - A test in which several electronic sensors are placed on the body to monitor electrical activity associated with the heartbeat.

Electroencephalogram (EEG) - A test that can detect and record the brain's electrical activity. The test is done by pasting metal disks, called electrodes, to the scalp.

Electrophysiological study (EPS) - A test that uses cardiac catheterization to study patients who have arrhythmias (abnormal heartbeats). An electrical current stimulates the heart in an effort to provoke an arrhythmia, determine its origin, and test the effectiveness of medicines to treat the arrhythmias.

Embolus - Also called embolism; a blood clot that forms in a blood vessel in one part of the body and travels to another part.

Endarterectomy - Surgical removal of plaque deposits or blood clots in an artery.

Endocardium - The smooth membrane covering the inside of the heart. The innermost lining of the heart.

Endothelium - The smooth inner lining of many body structures, including the heart (endocardium) and blood vessels.

Endocarditis - A bacterial infection of the heart's inner lining (endothelium).

Enlarged heart - A state in which the heart is larger than normal because of heredity, long-term heavy exercise, or diseases and disorders such as obesity, high blood pressure, and coronary artery disease.

Enzyme - A complex chemical capable of speeding up specific biochemical processes in the body.

Epicardium - The thin membrane covering the outside surface of the heart muscle.

Estrogen - A female hormone produced by the ovaries that may protect premenopausal women against heart disease. Estrogen production stops after menopause.

Estrogen (or hormone) replacement therapy (ERT or HRT) - Hormones that some women may take to offset the effects of menopause.

Exercise stress test - A common test to help doctors assess blood flow through coronary arteries in response to exercise, usually walking, at varied speeds and for various lengths of time on a treadmill. A stress test may include use of electrocardiography, echocardiography, and injected radioactive substances. Also called exercise test, stress test, nuclear stress test, or treadmill test.

Familial hypercholesterolemia - A genetic predisposition to dangerously high cholesterol levels.

Fatty acids (fats) - Substances that occur in several forms in foods; different fatty acids have different effects on lipid profiles.

Fibrillation - Rapid, uncoordinated contractions of individual heart muscle fibers. The heart chamber involved can't contract all at once and pumps blood ineffectively, if at all.

First-degree heart block - Occurs when an electrical impulse from the heart's upper chambers (the atria) is slowed as it moves through the atria and atrioventricular (AV) node.

Flutter - The rapid, ineffective contractions of any heart chamber. A flutter is considered to be more coordinated than fibrillation.

Fusiform aneurysm - A tube-shaped aneurysm that causes the artery to bulge outward. Involves the entire circumference (outside wall) of the artery.

Gated blood pool scan - An x-ray analysis of how blood pools in the heart during rest and exercise. The test uses a radioactive substance to tag red blood cells to allow doctors to estimate the heart's overall ability to pump and its ability to compensate for one or more blocked arteries.

Also called MUGA (multiple gated acquisition scan) or nuclear ventriculography.

Genetic testing - Blood tests that study a person's genes to find out if he or she is at risk for certain diseases that are passed down through family members.

Guidewire - A small, bendable wire that is threaded through an artery; it helps doctors position a catheter so they can perform angioplasty or stent procedures.

Heart assist device - A mechanical device that is surgically implanted to ease the workload of the heart.

Heart attack - Death of, or damage to, part of the heart muscle caused by a lack of oxygen-rich blood flowing to the heart.

Heart block - General term for conditions in which the electrical impulse that activates the heart muscle cells is delayed or interrupted somewhere along its path.

Heart failure - See congestive heart failure.

Heart-lung machine - An apparatus that oxygenates and pumps blood to the body during open heart surgery; see cardiopulmonary bypass.

Heart murmur -An abnormal heart sound caused by turbulent blood flow. The sound may indicate that blood is flowing through a damaged or overworked heart valve, that there may be a hole in one of the heart's walls, or that there is a narrowing in one of the heart's vessels. Some heart murmurs are a harmless type called innocent heart murmurs.

Hematocrit - A measure of the percentage of red blood cells in a given amount (or volume) of whole blood.

Hemochromatosis - A disease in which too much iron builds up in your body (iron overload). Too much iron in the heart can cause irregular heartbeats (arrhythmias) and heart failure. Too much iron in the pancreas can lead to diabetes.

Heredity - The genetic transmission of a particular quality or trait from parent to child.

High blood pressure - A chronic increase in blood pressure above its normal range.

High density lipoprotein (HDL) - A component of cholesterol, HDL helps protect against heart disease by promoting cholesterol breakdown and removal from the blood; hence, its nickname "good cholesterol."

Holter monitor - A portable device for recording heartbeats over a period of 24 hours or more.

Homocysteine – An amino acid (one of the building blocks that makes up a protein) normally found in small amounts in the blood. Too much homocysteine in the blood may promote the buildup of fatty plaque in the arteries. For some people, high homocysteine levels are genetic. For others, it is because they do not get enough of certain B vitamins in their diet. (Common misspelling: homocystine)

Hormones - Chemicals released into the bloodstream that control different functions in the body, including metabolism, growth, sexual development, and responses to stress or illness.

Hypertension - High blood pressure.

Hypertrophic obstructive cardiomyopathy (HOCM) - An overgrown heart muscle that creates a bulge into the ventricle and impedes blood flow.

Hypertrophy - Enlargement of tissues or organs because of increased workload.

Hyperventilation - Rapid breathing usually caused by anxiety. People feel like they can't get enough air, so they breathe heavily and rapidly, which can lead to numb or tingly arms and legs, or fainting.

Hypoglycemia - Low levels of glucose (sugar) in the blood.

Hypokinesia - Decreased muscle movement. In relation to the heart, hypokinesia refers to decreased heart wall motion during each heartbeat. It is associated with cardiomyopathy, heart failure, or heart attack. Also called hypokinesis.

Hypotension - Abnormally low blood pressure.

Hypoxia - Less than normal content of oxygen in the organs and tissues of the body.

Idiopathic - No known cause.

Immunosuppressants - Any medicine that suppresses the body's immune system. These medicines are used to minimize the chances that the body will reject a newly transplanted organ, such as a heart.

Impedance plethysmography - A noninvasive diagnostic test used to evaluate blood flow through the leg.

Incompetent valve - Also called insufficiency; a valve that is not working properly, causing it to leak blood back in the wrong direction.

Infarct - The area of heart tissue permanently damaged by an inadequate supply of oxygen.

Infective endocarditis - An infection of the heart valves and the innermost lining of the heart (the endocardium), caused by bacteria in the bloodstream.

Inferior vena cava - The large vein returning blood from the legs and abdomen to the heart.

Inotropes - Positive inotropes: Any medicine that increases the strength of the heart's contraction. Negative inotropes: Any medicine that decreases the strength of the heart's contraction and the blood pressure in the vessels.

Internal mammary artery - A durable artery in the chest wall often used as a bypass graft in coronary artery bypass surgery.

Intravascular echocardiography - A combination of echocardiography and cardiac catheterization. A miniature echo device on the tip of a catheter is used to generate images inside the heart and blood vessels.

Introducer sheath - A catheter-like tube that is placed inside a patient's vessel during an interventional procedure to help the doctor with insertion and proper placement of the actual catheter.

Ischemia - Decreased blood flow to an organ, usually due to constriction or obstruction of an artery.

Ischemic heart disease - Also called coronary artery disease and coronary heart disease, this term is applied to heart problems caused by narrowing of the coronary arteries, thereby causing a decreased blood supply to the heart.

Ischemic stroke - A type of stroke that is caused by blockage in a blood vessel.

Jugular veins - The veins that carry blood back from the head to the heart.

Left ventricular assist device (LVAD) - A mechanical device that can be placed outside the body or implanted inside the body. An LVAD does not replace the heart—it "assists" or "helps" it pump oxygen-rich blood from the left ventricle to the rest of the body.

Lesion - An injury or wound. An atherosclerotic lesion is an injury to an artery due to hardening of the arteries.

Lipid - A fatty substance that is insoluble (cannot be dissolved) in the blood.

Lipoprotein - A lipid surrounded by a protein; the protein makes the lipid soluble (can be dissolved) in the blood.

Low density lipoprotein (LDL) - The body's primary cholesterol-carrying molecule. High blood levels of LDL increase a person's risk of heart disease by promoting cholesterol attachment and accumulation in blood vessels; hence, the popular nickname "bad cholesterol."

Lumen - The hollow area within a tube, such as a blood vessel.

Magnetic resonance imaging (MRI) - A technique that produces images of the heart and other body structures by measuring the response of certain elements (such as hydrogen) in the body to a magnetic field. MRI can produce detailed pictures of the heart and its various structures without the need to inject a dye.

Maze surgery - A type of heart surgery that is used to treat chronic atrial fibrillation by creating a surgical "maze" of new electrical pathways to let electrical impulses travel easily through the heart. Also called the Maze procedure.

Mitral stenosis - A narrowing of the mitral valve, which controls blood flow from the heart's upper left chamber to its lower left chamber. May result from an inherited (congenital) problem or from rheumatic fever.

Mitral valve - The structure that controls blood flow between the heart's left atrium (upper chamber) and left ventricle (lower chamber).

Mitral valve prolapse - A condition that occurs when the leaflets of the mitral valve between the left atrium and left ventricle bulge into the atrium and permit backflow of blood. The condition can be associated with progressive mitral regurgitation.

Mitral valve regurgitation - Failure of the mitral valve to close properly, causing blood to flow back into the heart's upper left chamber (the left atrium) instead of moving forward into the lower left chamber (the left ventricle).

mm Hg - An abbreviation for millimeters of mercury. Blood pressure is measured in units of mm Hg—how high the pressure inside the arteries would be able to raise a column of mercury.

Monounsaturated fats - A type of fat found in many foods but mainly in avocados and in canola, olive, and peanut oils. Monounsaturated fat tends to lower LDL cholesterol levels, and some studies suggest that it may do so without also lowering HDL cholesterol levels.

Mortality - The total number of deaths from a given disease in a population during an interval of time, usually a year.

Murmur - Noises superimposed on normal heart sounds. They are caused by congenital defects or damaged heart valves that do not close properly and allow blood to leak back into the chamber from which it has come.

Myocardial infarction - A heart attack. The damage or death of an area of the heart muscle (myocardium) resulting from a blocked blood supply to the area. The affected tissue dies, injuring the heart. Symptoms include prolonged, intensive chest pain and a decrease in blood pressure that often causes shock.

Myocardial ischemia - Occurs when a part of the heart muscle does not receive enough oxygen.

Myocarditis – A rare condition in which the heart muscle becomes inflamed as a result of infection, toxic drug poisoning, or diseases like rheumatic fever, diphtheria, or tuberculosis.

Myocardium - The muscular wall of the heart. It contracts to pump blood out of the heart and then relaxes as the heart refills with returning blood.

Myxomatous degeneration - A connective tissue disorder that causes the heart valve tissue to weaken and lose elasticity.

Nitroglycerin - A medicine that helps relax and dilate arteries; often used to treat cardiac chest pain (angina).

Necrosis - Refers to the death of tissue within a certain area.

Noninvasive procedures - Any diagnostic or treatment procedure in which no instrument enters the body.

NSTEMI - Non-ST-segment-elevation myocardial infarction. The milder form of the 2 types of heart attack, an NSTEMI does not produce an ST-segment elevation on an electrocardiogram. See also STEMI.

Obesity - The condition of being significantly overweight. It usually applies when a person is 30% or more over ideal body weight. Obesity puts a strain on the heart and can increase the risk of developing high blood pressure and diabetes.

Occluded artery - An artery in which the blood flow has been impaired by a blockage.

Open heart surgery - An operation in which the chest and heart are opened surgically while the bloodstream is diverted through a heart-lung (cardiopulmonary bypass) machine.

Pacemaker - A surgically implanted electronic device that helps regulate the heartbeat.

Palpitation - An uncomfortable feeling within the chest caused by an irregular heartbeat.

Pancreas - The organ behind the stomach that helps control blood sugar levels.

Pancreatitis - Swelling (inflammation) of the pancreas.

Paralysis -Loss of the ability to move muscles and feel in part of the body or the whole body. Paralysis may be temporary or permanent.

Paroxysmal supraventricular tachycardia (PSVT) – An occasional rapid heart rate (150-250 beats per minute) that is caused by events triggered in areas above the heart's lower chambers (the ventricles). See also supraventricular tachycardia (SVT).

Patent ductus arteriosus - A congenital defect in which the opening between the aorta and the pulmonary artery does not close after birth.

Patent foramen ovale - An opening between the left and right atria (the upper chambers) of the heart. Everyone has a PFO before birth, but in 1 out of every 3 or 4 people, the opening does not close naturally, as it should, after birth.

Percutaneous coronary intervention (PCI) - Any of the noninvasive procedures usually performed in the cardiac catheterization laboratory. Angioplasty is an example of a percutaneous coronary intervention. Also called a transcatheter intervention.

Percutaneous transluminal coronary angioplasty (PTCA) - See angioplasty.

Pericarditis - Inflammation of the outer membrane surrounding the heart. When pericarditis occurs, the amount of fluid between the two layers of the pericardium increases. This increased fluid presses on the heart and restricts its pumping action.

Pericardiocentesis - A diagnostic procedure that uses a needle to withdraw fluid from the sac or membrane surrounding the heart (pericardium).

Pericardium - The outer fibrous sac that surrounds the heart.

Plaque - A deposit of fatty (and other) substances in the inner lining of the artery wall characteristic of atherosclerosis.

Platelets - One of the three types of cells found in blood; they aid in the clotting of blood.

Polyunsaturated fat - The major fat in most vegetable oils, including corn, safflower, sunflower, and soybean oils. These oils are liquid at room temperature. Polyunsaturated fat actually tends to lower LDL cholesterol levels but may reduce HDL cholesterol levels as well.

Positron emission tomography (PET) - A test that uses information about the energy of certain elements in your body to show whether parts of the heart muscle are alive and working. A PET scan can also show if your heart is getting enough blood to keep the muscle healthy.

Postural orthostatic tachycardia syndrome (POTS) - A disorder that causes an increased heart rate when a person stands upright.

Premature ventricular contraction (PVC) - An early or extra heartbeat that happens when the heart's lower chambers (the ventricles) contract too soon, out of sequence with the normal heartbeat.

Prevalence - The total number of cases of a given disease that exist in a population at a specific time.

Pulmonary - Refers to the lungs and respiratory system.

Pulmonary embolism - A condition in which a blood clot that has formed elsewhere in the body travels to the lungs.

Pulmonary valve - The heart valve between the right ventricle and the pulmonary artery that controls blood flow from the heart into the lungs.

Pulmonary vein - The blood vessel that carries newly oxygenated blood from the lungs back to the left atrium of the heart.

Radial artery access - Using the radial artery in the wrist as the entry point for the catheter in an angioplasty or stent procedure. Also called transradial access, the transradial approach, or transradial angioplasty.

Radionuclide imaging - A test in which a harmless radioactive substance is injected into the bloodstream to show information about blood flow through the arteries. Damaged or dead heart muscle can often be identified, as can serious narrowing in an artery.

Radionuclide studies - Any of the diagnostic tests in which a small amount of radioactive material is injected into the bloodstream. The material makes it possible for a special camera to take pictures of the heart.

Radionuclide ventriculography - A diagnostic test used to determine the size and shape of the heart's pumping chambers (the ventricles).

Regurgitation - Backward flow of blood through a defective heart valve.

Renal - Pertains to the kidneys.

Restenosis- The re-closing or re-narrowing of an artery after an interventional procedure such as angioplasty or stent placement.

Revascularization - A procedure to restore blood flow to the tissues. Coronary artery bypass surgery is an example of a revascularization procedure.

Rheumatic fever - A disease, usually occurring in childhood that may follow a streptococcal infection. Symptoms may include fever, sore or swollen joints, skin rash, involuntary muscle twitching, and development of nodules under the skin. If the infection involves the heart, scars may form on heart valves, and the heart's outer lining may be damaged.

Rheumatic heart disease - A disease of the heart (mainly affecting the heart valves) caused by rheumatic fever.

Right ventricular assist device (RVAD) - A mechanical device that can be placed outside the body or implanted inside the body. An RVAD does not replace the heart—it "assists" or "helps" it pump oxygen-poor blood from the right ventricle to the lungs.

Risk factor - An element or condition involving a certain hazard or danger. When referring to heart and blood vessels, a risk factor is associated with an increased chance of developing cardiovascular disease, including stroke.

Rubella - Commonly known as German measles.

Saccular aneurysm - A round aneurysm that bulges out from an artery; involves only part of the circumference (outside wall) of the artery.

Sarcoidosis - An inflammatory disease that starts as tiny, grain-like lumps called granulomas, which most often appear in your lungs or lymph nodes. The granulomas can clump together and form larger lumps that attack other organs. Sarcoidosis often affects your skin, eyes, or liver, but it can lead to heart problems, such as irregular heartbeats (arrhythmias) or restrictive cardiomyopathy.

Saturated fat - Type of fat found in foods of animal origin and a few of vegetable origin; they are usually solid at room temperature. Abundant in meat and dairy products, saturated fat tends to increase LDL cholesterol levels, and it may raise the risk of certain types of cancer.

Second-degree heart block - Impulses traveling through the heart's upper chambers (the atria) are delayed in the area between the upper and lower chambers (the AV node) and fail to make the ventricles beat at the right moment.

Septal defect - A hole in the wall of the heart separating the atria or in the wall of the heart separating the ventricles.

Septum - The muscular wall dividing a chamber on the left side of the heart from the chamber on the right.

Sheath - A catheter-like tube that is placed inside a patient's vessel during an interventional procedure to help the doctor with insertion and proper placement of the actual catheter. Also called an introducer sheath.

Shock - A condition in which body function is impaired because the volume of fluid circulating through the body is insufficient to maintain normal metabolism. This may be caused by blood loss or by a disturbance in the function of the circulatory system.

Shunt - A connector that allows blood to flow between two locations.

Sick sinus syndrome - The failure of the sinus node to regulate the heart's rhythm.

Silent ischemia - Episodes of cardiac ischemia that are not accompanied by chest pain.

Sinus (SA) node - The "natural" pacemaker of the heart. The node is a group of specialized cells in the top of the right atrium which produces the electrical impulses that travel down to eventually reach the ventricular muscle, causing the heart to contract.

Sodium - A mineral essential to life found in nearly all plant and animal tissue. Table salt (sodium chloride) is nearly half sodium.

Sphygmomanometer - An instrument used to measure blood pressure.

Stem cells - Special cells in the body that are able to transform into other cells. It is possible for stem cells to transform into heart cells, nerve cells, or other cells of the body, possibly helping to improve the function of failing organs, including the heart.

STEMI - ST-segment-elevation myocardial infarction. The more severe form of the 2 types of heart attack. See also NSTEMI. A STEMI produces a characteristic elevation in the ST segment on an electrocardiogram.

Stent - A device made of expandable, metal mesh that is placed (by using a balloon catheter) at the site of a narrowing artery. The stent is then expanded and left in place to keep the artery open.

Stenosis - The narrowing or constriction of an opening, such as a blood vessel or heart valve.

Stethoscope - An instrument for listening to sounds within the body.

Stokes-Adams disease - Also called third-degree heart block; a condition that happens when the impulses that pace your heartbeat do not reach the lower chambers of your heart (the ventricles). To make up for this, the ventricles use their own "backup" pacemaker with its slower rate. This rhythm can cause severe dizziness or fainting and can lead to heart failure or death.

Streptococcal infection ("strep" infection) - An infection, usually in the throat, resulting from the presence of streptococcus bacteria.

Streptokinase - A clot-dissolving medicine used to treat heart attack patients.

Sternum - The breastbone.

Stress - Bodily or mental tension resulting from physical, chemical, or emotional factors. Stress can refer to physical exertion as well as mental anxiety.

Stroke - A sudden disruption of blood flow to the brain, either by a clot or a leak in a blood vessel.

Subarachnoid hemorrhage - Bleeding from a blood vessel on the surface of the brain into the space between the brain and the skull.

Subclavian arteries - Two major arteries (right and left) that receive blood from the aortic arch and supply it to the arms.

Sudden death - Death that occurs unexpectedly and instantaneously or shortly after the onset of symptoms. The most common underlying reason for patients dying suddenly is cardiovascular disease, in particular coronary heart disease.

Superior vena cava - The large vein that returns blood from the head and arms to the heart.

Supraventricular tachycardia (SVT) - A regular rapid heart rate (150-250 beats per minute) that is caused by events triggered in areas above the heart's lower chambers (the ventricles); see also paroxysmal supraventricular tachycardia (PSVT).

Syncope - A temporary, insufficient blood supply to the brain which causes a loss of consciousness. Usually caused by a serious arrhythmia.

Systolic blood pressure - The highest blood pressure measured in the arteries. It occurs when the heart contracts with each heartbeat.

Tachycardia - Accelerated beating of the heart. Paroxysmal tachycardia is a particular form of rapid heart action, occurring in seizures that may last from a few seconds to several days.

Tachypnea - Rapid breathing.

Tamponade - Also called cardiac tamponade. A condition in which the heart is compressed or constricted because of a large amount of fluid or blood in the space between the heart muscle and the sac that surrounds the heart (the pericardium).

Thallium-201 stress test - An x-ray study that follows the path of radioactive potassium carried by the blood into heart muscle. Damaged or dead muscle can be defined, as can the extent of narrowing in an artery.

Third-degree heart block - A serious condition also called Stokes-Adams disease; impulses from the heart's upper chambers (the atria) are completely blocked from reaching the heart's lower chambers (the ventricles). To make up for this, the ventricles use their own "backup" pacemaker with its slower rate.

Thrombolysis - The breaking up of a blood clot.

Thrombosis - A blood clot that forms inside the blood vessel or cavity of the heart.

Thrombolytic therapy - Intravenous or intra-arterial medicines that are used to dissolve blood clots in an artery.

Thrombus - A blood clot.

Thyroid - A gland located in the front of the neck, just below the voice box.

Tissue plasminogen activator (tPA) - A clot-dissolving medicine that is used to treat heart attack and stroke patients.

Trans fat - Created when hydrogen is forced through an ordinary vegetable oil (hydrogenation), converting some polyunsaturates to monounsaturates, and some monounsaturates to saturates. Trans fat, like saturated fat, tends to raise LDL cholesterol levels, and, unlike saturated fat, trans fat also lowers HDL cholesterol levels.

Transcatheter aortic valve implantation (TAVI) - A minimally invasive procedure to repair a damaged or diseased aortic valve. A catheter is inserted into an artery in the groin and threaded to the heart. A balloon at the end of the catheter, with a replacement valve folded around it, delivers the new valve to take the place of the old. Also called TAVR (Tran's catheter aortic valve replacement).

Transcatheter intervention - Any of the noninvasive procedures usually performed in the cardiac catheterization laboratory. Angioplasty is an example of a transcatheter intervention. Also called a percutaneous coronary intervention (PCI).

Transesophageal echocardiography - A diagnostic test that analyzes sound waves bounced off the heart. The sound waves are sent through a tube-like device inserted in the mouth and passed down the esophagus (food pipe), which ends near the heart. This technique is useful in studying patients whose heart and vessels, for various reasons, are difficult to assess with standard echocardiography.

Transient ischemic attack (TIA) - A stroke-like event that lasts only for a short time and is caused by a temporarily blocked blood vessel.

Transplantation - Replacing a failing organ with a healthy one from a donor.

Tricuspid valve - The structure that controls blood flow from the heart's upper right chamber (the right atrium) into the lower right chamber (the right ventricle).

Triglyceride - The most common fatty substance found in the blood; normally stored as an energy source in fat tissue. High triglyceride levels may thicken the blood and make a person more susceptible to clot formation. High triglyceride levels tend to accompany high cholesterol levels and other risk factors for heart disease, such as obesity.

Ultrasound - High-frequency sound vibrations, which cannot be heard by the human ear, used in medical diagnosis.

Valve replacement - An operation to replace a heart valve that is either blocking normal blood flow or causing blood to leak backward into the heart (regurgitation).

Valvuloplasty - Reshaping of a heart valve with surgical or catheter techniques.

Varicose vein - Any vein that is abnormally dilated (widened).

Vascular - Pertains to the blood vessels.

Vasodilators - Any medicine that dilates (widens) the arteries.

Vasopressors - Any medicine that elevates blood pressure.

Vein - Any one of a series of blood vessels of the vascular system that carries blood from various parts of the body back to the heart, returning oxygen-poor blood to the heart.

Ventricle (right and left) - One of the two lower chambers of the heart.

Ventricular Assist Device (VAD) - A mechanical pump that helps the ventricles pump blood, easing the workload of the heart in patients with heart failure.

Ventricular fibrillation - A condition in which the ventricles contract in a rapid, unsynchronized fashion. When fibrillation occurs, the ventricles cannot pump blood throughout the body.

Ventricular tachycardia - An arrhythmia (abnormal heartbeat) in the ventricle characterized by a very fast heartbeat.

Vertigo - A feeling of dizziness or spinning.

Wolff-Parkinson-White syndrome - A condition in which an extra electrical pathway connects the atria (two upper chambers) and the ventricles (two lower chambers). It may cause a rapid heartbeat.

X-ray - Form of radiation used to create a picture of internal body structures on film.

EQUIPMENT STERILIZATION

INTRODUCTION

Following established protocols, i.e., best practices for instrument reprocessing is an important aspect of modern health care as it helps to minimize the patient's risk of infection. This article is intended to provide an overview of the six (6) recommended steps for instrument reprocessing; cleaning, inspection, packaging, sterilization, sterile storage, and quality assurance.

STEP 1: CLEANING

The first and most important step in instrument reprocessing is cleaning, as studies [Alfa, 1998] have shown that a dirty instrument cannot be effectively sterilized. This is because the soil shields bacteria and viruses from the sterilizing agent. As a result, bacteria and viruses may very well survive the sterilization process and can cross infect the next patient.

The most common method of cleaning instruments is manual cleaning (cleaning by hand). Manual cleaning has the advantage of flexibility, in that any type of instrument can be cleaned manually. Drawbacks to manual cleaning are that the cleanliness of the instruments can vary between workers as well as that employees are at risk of being exposed to possible cross infection as they are in contact with contaminated instruments. For these reasons, it is important that health care facilities establish protocols for instrument cleaning and require staff to wear proper personal protection equipment (PPE) when working with contaminated instruments.

Recommended procedures for manual cleaning are to first soak the instrument in a tepid or lukewarm water or detergent bath for at least 10 minutes. This step softens and loosens much of the soil that may have dried on the instrument between the time it was used and the time cleaning has started. The duration of the soak depends upon how much soil is on the instruments and how long the soil has been allowed to dry. Note: The use of enzyme detergents is preferred as they help to break up organic soil more readily and rapidly than do conventional detergents. The next step is to completely brush the instrument with a medium-soft bristle brush while it is in the soak bath. In the case of tubed devices like dental hand pieces, the insides (lumens, channels, etc.) should be brushed out as well. Care should be taken to use brushes recommended by the manufacturer to avoid damaging the instrument. Note: Brushing should be done under the surface of the water to minimize aerosols and with brush strokes away from the body to avoid exposure to spray from the brush. The instrument should then be rinsed with clean water and, if difficult-to-remove soil remains, another enzyme soak followed by brushing and rinsing should be done.

Ultrasonic Cleaning
For health care facilities that have them, ultrasonic cleaning is a great follow-up to manual cleaning. Although manual cleaning removes most or all of the visible soil from instruments, it may not remove small or microscopic particles that are protected by the texture of a surface or design features like hinges. Ultrasonic cleaners create microscopic bubbles in the solution that

collapse when they contact the instrument releasing energy. This energy "kicks" any soil that is in the area off the instrument. This process is called cavitation. The detergent in the ultrasonic bath suspends the soil particles and keeps them from attaching back to the instruments. Ultrasonic cleaning should be done for a duration specified by the instrument, detergent, or ultrasonic bath manufacturer, whichever is longer. Following ultrasonic cleaning, the instruments are rinsed with clean water and dried. Distilled water is preferred to ensure removal of as much detergent as possible but is only essential if the tap water has a high mineral content that could cause spotting. After drying, the instruments may be packaged for sterilization.

Automatic Washers
Practices that need to clean a large quantity of instruments and/or cassettes should consider purchasing automatic cleaning machines. These machines may resemble home dishwashers or be specialized for the specific needs of cleaning complex instruments, e.g., endoscopic instruments. Validated to meet the special needs of cleaning instruments, automatic washers offer a wide range of temperature settings that allow the instruments to be processed at the maximum safe temperature for their use. Higher temperatures speed cleaning and provide some disinfection. Regardless of the automatic washer type used, instruments must be prepared for processing before being placed into a washer, with the extent of preparation depending upon the capabilities of the washer. The actual preparation must be done in accordance with the washer manufacturer's instructions. For the simplest washers, manual presoaking and sonication remain as necessary reprocessing steps. More sophisticated washers include a presoaking step in the automated process.

STEP 2: INSPECTION

Each and every instrument should be inspected for function and cleanliness after cleaning. Any damaged instrument should be replaced and any instrument with visible soil or residual debris should be returned for further cleaning. Never clean a dirty instrument in a clean area unless you have proper PPE. The cleaning action can cross contaminate other instruments and work surfaces. Special Note: Instruments with stiff joints may be a sign of inadequate cleaning.

STEP 3: PACKAGING

Sterile packaging, i.e., pouches, wrap, or rigid containers serve to maintain the sterility of processed instruments and allow for aseptic opening at point of use. Packaging should be done in a clean area using FDA-cleared materials such as pouches, wrap, or rigid containers.

Pouches
Sterilization pouches are commonly used for small, lightweight instruments and should be placed on edge facing the same direction in the sterilizer. This best practice loading technique assists sterility penetration and facilitates drying. Prior to sealing a sterilization pouch, it is important to include a "multiparameter" chemical indicator and remove excess air. With self-sealing pouches, be sure to fold the adhesive flap on the perforation line and make contact with both the paper and plastic film (ideally 50% each). Some sterilization pouches come printed with both external and internal chemical indicators. This complies with CDC guidelines, providing the supplier has

validated the internal indicator as a multiparameter indicator.

Wrap
Sterilization wrap is commonly used for instrument trays or cassettes. There are many different types and sizes of wraps available. Typically, two sheets are needed to provide an effective barrier and a specific technique is recommended [CDC, AAMI ST79] to allow for aseptic opening. Wrapped instruments should be secured with sterilization tape that also serves as an external indicator. Before closing, a multi-parameter chemical indicator should be included inside along with the instruments. Be sure to select the correct size wrap and be careful not to wrap too tight or too loose as either can compromise sterility by creating air pockets or allowing strike through. Recently, wrap manufacturers have stated not to stack wrapped items during storage as this can compromise sterility.

Rigid Containers
Sterilization containers are commonly used for heavy, mostly layered instrument trays, i.e., orthopedic sets. A maximum weight of 25 pounds has been established [AAMI ST79, AORN] regardless of the instrument trays being wrapped or placed in rigid containers. There are many different types and sizes of rigid containers, all of which provide excellent protection during storage and can be stacked during storage without compromising sterility. For quality assurance, a multiparameter chemical indicator should be included on each layer of multilayered sets and in opposite corners of rigid containers.

STEP 4: STERILIZATION

Steam sterilization is the most commonly used process for sterilizing instruments, trays, and cassettes. According to the CDC, steam under pressure is the process of choice whenever possible as it is considered safe, fast, and the most cost-effective for health care facilities. Steam sterilizers come in many different sizes and sterilizer cycles can vary among manufacturers. The cycle a sterilizer runs can typically be found in the sterilizer manual. The following are examples of standard cycle parameters (AAMI ST79, AORN) for packaged instruments.

Gravity – 121°C/250°F for 30 minutes exposure and 15–30 minutes drying time

Gravity – 132°C/270°F for 15 minutes exposure and 15–30 minutes drying time

Gravity – 135°C/275°F for 10 minutes exposure and 30 minutes drying time

Dynamic Air Removal – 132°C/270°F for 4 minutes exposure and 20–30 minutes drying time

Dynamic Air Removal – 135°C/275°F for 3 minutes exposure and 16 minutes drying time

Other commercially available sterilization processes include: chemical vapor, dry heat, ethylene oxide, vaporized hydrogen peroxide, and ozone. Although each of these processes offer advantages and disadvantages, the decision about which sterilization process the health care facility should choose lies with the instrument manufacturer as to what was validated in their instructions for use (IFU). For patient safety, the process must be compatible as to not cause damage and must be efficacious to ensure sterility.

STEP 5: STERILE STORAGE

Sterilized packages should be stored in a manner that reduces the potential for contamination, i.e., clean, dry, and temperature- and traffic-controlled areas. Sterility is event related and sterile items are considered sterile unless damaged or open. Therefore, it is important for sterilized packages to be handled with care: avoid dragging, crushing, bending, compressing, or puncturing. During transport, they should be protected from environmental contaminants. Prior to use, each sterilized package should be inspected for integrity. If a package is suspect, it should not be used and the item should be reprocessed. Sterile packages should not be opened until point of use.

STEP 6: QUALITY ASSURANCE

Sterility assurance of processed instruments should be routinely verified using three (3) types of indicators; physical, chemical, and biological.

Physical Indicators
Physical indicators consist of the time, temperature, and pressure gauges built into sterilizers. For each sterilization cycle, these readings should be observed and verified prior to unloading the sterilizer. Large freestanding sterilizers, which are often found in surgery centers and hospitals, are required to have a chart or printout that is initialed after each cycle. This physical indicator is then maintained as part of their overall infection-control records. Many tabletop sterilizers do not provide physical indicator printouts.

Chemical Indicators
Chemical indicators (CIs) change color or show movement during the sterilizer cycle to verify that some or all sterilization parameters were met. As stated earlier, CIs should be used on the outside and inside of all sterilized packages. CIs range in performance characteristics and health care facilities should select the CI that best fits their monitoring needs. Indicator tape is an example of an external CI and it simply indicates that a package was run in the sterilizer. Internal CIs are used to ensure the sterilant penetrates the packaging system and a Class 5 integrating indicator demonstrates that ALL of the parameters necessary for sterilization were met for that specific cycle.

If using a dynamic air removal (pre-vacuum) sterilizer, an air removal test should be run daily. This is called a Bowie-Dick type test and passes when the chemical indicator sheet inside a process challenge device (PCD) changes to a uniform color after processing at 134°C/274°F for 3.5- or 4-minute exposure time. This test should be run in an empty sterilizer and drying time is optional as this daily air removal test is performed without a load.

Biological Indicators
Biological Indicator (BI) monitoring is the gold standard for sterility assurance [CDC, 2003,

2008] as BI's contain bacterial spores that test the lethality of sterilizers. The science behind this is, if your sterilizer can effectively kill the highly resistant spores in the BI, then we can be confident it is capable of killing the less resistant organisms found on our instruments. Biological Indicators are available in both mail-in and in-office systems. BIs should be run at least weekly, per CDC guidelines [CDC, 2003, 2008]. Weekly BI monitoring is completed by running a BI in the sterilizer with a load. In-office BI testing requires test vials, a preset incubator, and a record notebook. After processing, the BI is incubated at a preset.

SURGICAL INSTRUMENTS

A **surgical instrument** is a specially designed tool or device for performing specific actions of carrying out desired effects during a surgery or operation, such as modifying biological tissue or to provide access for viewing it. Over time, many different kinds of surgical instruments and tools have been invented. Some surgical instruments are designed for general use in surgery, while others are designed for a specific procedure or surgery. Accordingly, the nomenclature of surgical instruments follows certain patterns, such as a description of the action it performs (for example, scalpel), the name of its inventor(s) (for example, the Kocher forceps), or a compound scientific name related to the kind of surgery (for example, a tracheotome is a tool used to perform a tracheotomy).

The expression **surgical instrumentation** is somewhat interchangeably used with surgical instruments, but its meaning in medical jargon is really the activity of providing assistance to a surgeon with the proper handling of surgical instruments during an operation, by a specialized professional, usually a Surgical technologist or sometimes a Nurse or radiographer.

History

Surgical instruments have been manufactured since the dawn of pre-history. Rough trephines for performing round craniotomies were discovered in Neolithic sites in many places. It is believed that they were used by shamans to release evil spirits and alleviate headaches and head traumas caused by war-inflicted wounds.

In the Antiquity, surgeons and physicians in Greece and Rome developed many ingenious instruments manufactured from bronze, iron and silver, such as scalpels, lancets, curettes, tweezers, speculae, trephines, forceps, probes, dilators, tubes, surgical knifes, etc. They are still very well preserved in several medical museums around the world. Most of these instruments continued to be used in Medieval times, albeit with a better manufacturing technique.

In the Renaissance and post-Renaissance era, new instruments were again invented and designed, in order to accompany the increased audacity of surgeons. Amputation sets originated in this period, due to the increased severity of war-inflicted wounds by shot, grapnel and cannon.

However, it was only with the discovery of anesthesia and surgical asepsis that new surgical instruments were invented to allow the penetration of the inner sanctum, or the previously forbidden body cavities, namely the skull, the thorax and the abdomen. A veritable explosion of new tools occurred with the hundreds of new surgical procedures which were developed in the 19th century and first decades of the 20th century. New materials, such as stainless steel, chrome, titanium and vanadium were available for the manufacturing of these instruments. Precision instruments for microsurgery in neurosurgery, ophthalmology and otology were possible and, in the second half of the 20th century, energy-based instruments were first developed, such as electrocauteries, ultrasound and electric scalpels, surgical tools for endoscopic surgery, and finally, surgical robots.

ABDOMINAL RETRACTORS

Common Uses:

Abdominal Retractors used to actively separate the edges of a surgical incision in abdomen. Abdominal retractors are self-retaining; they hold back underlying organs and tissues, so that body parts under the incision may be accessed.

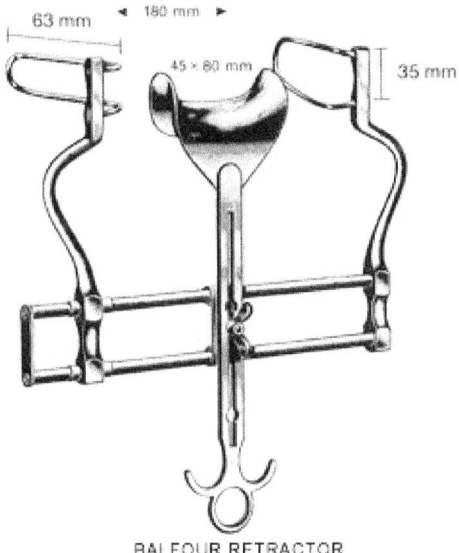

BALFOUR RETRACTOR

ANESTHESIA

Common Uses:

A laryngoscope is a medical device that is used to obtain a view of the vocal folds and the glottis which is the space between the cords.

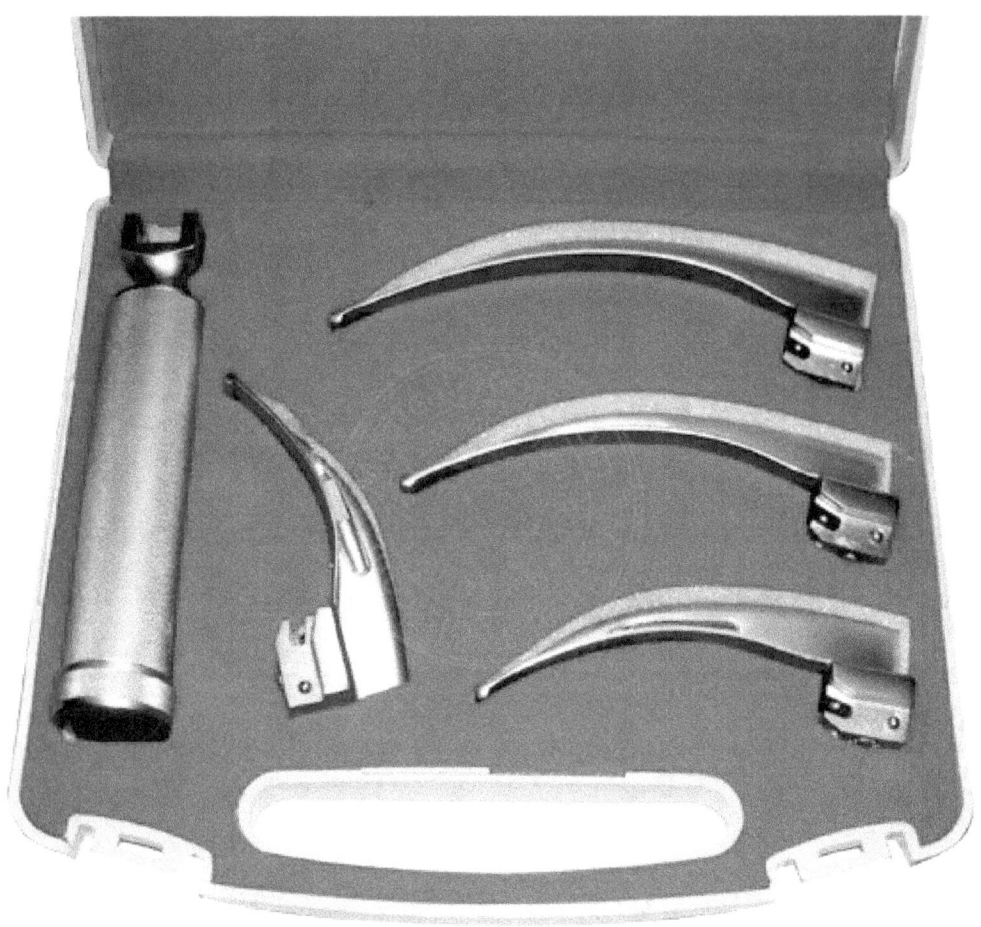

SPECIMEN FORCEPS

Common Uses:

Biopsy Forceps is an instrument to take a sample (bite) off the face of the cervix or from the edge of the cervical os (opening). This is done usually when the physician is suspicious of carcinoma (cancer) growing on the cervix. The sample is put into a vial of sterile saline and sent to the lab for analysis

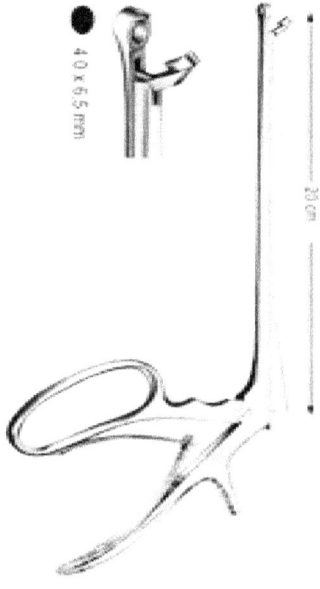

DISSECTING FORCEPS

Common Uses:
A wide range of dissecting forceps is available in different sizes. Medical Tools dissecting forceps feature fine serrations with precision points matching and ridges for better grip, excellent quality used by professionals.

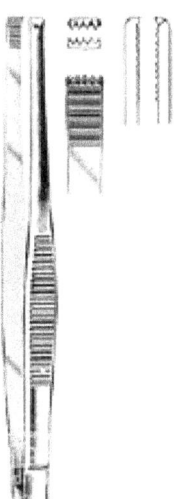

DRESSING FORCEPS

Common Uses:

Dressing Forceps are used to hold swabs or sponges for mopping up the site.

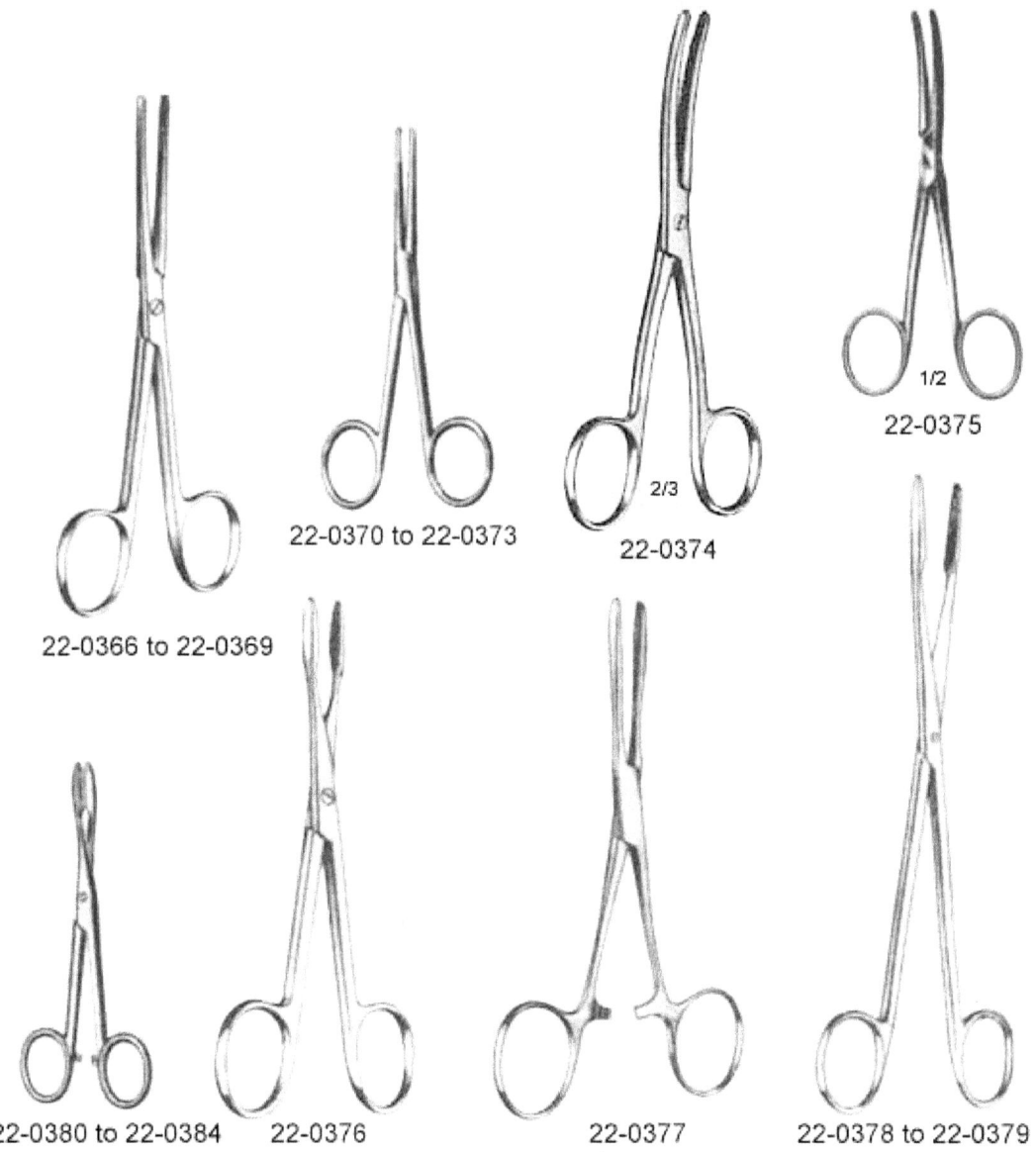

MOUTH AND TONGUE

Common Uses:

Mouth and tongue instruments are used in oral and ENT procedures. Mouth gags are used to retain mouth opening open during procedure while cheek lip and tongue retractors are also be used to facilitate procedure.

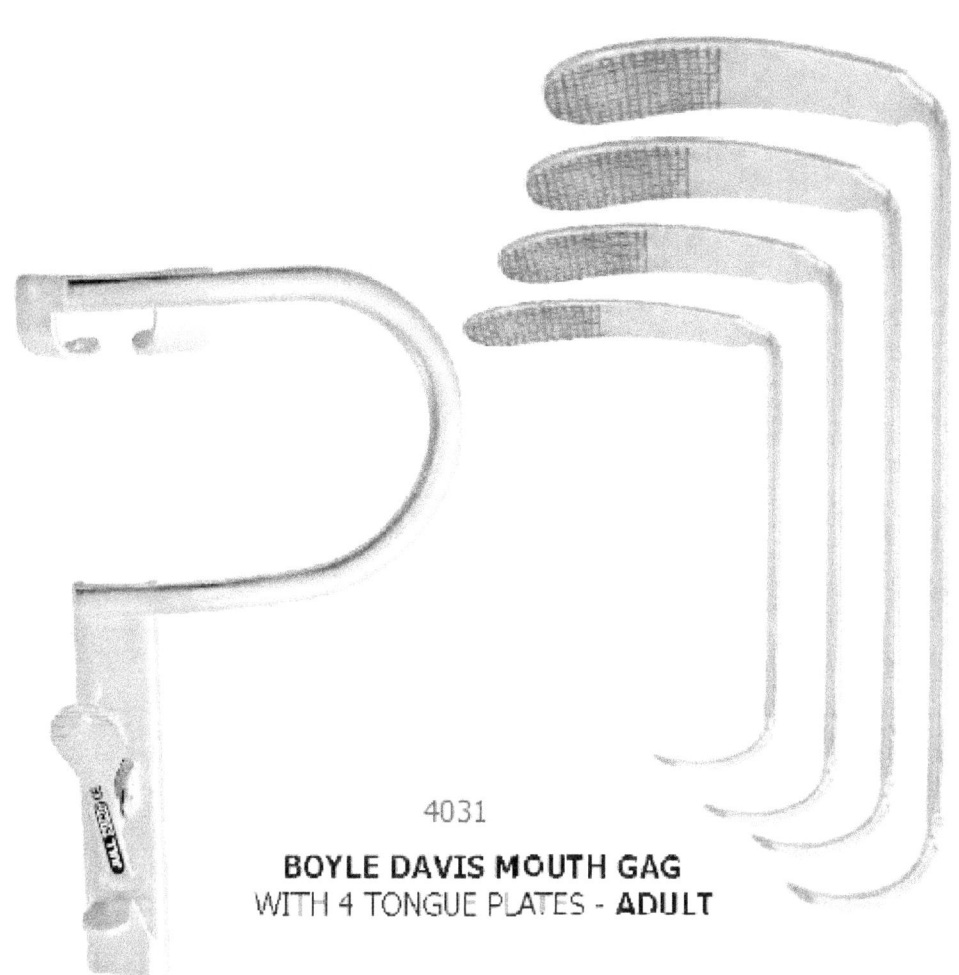

4031

BOYLE DAVIS MOUTH GAG
WITH 4 TONGUE PLATES - **ADULT**

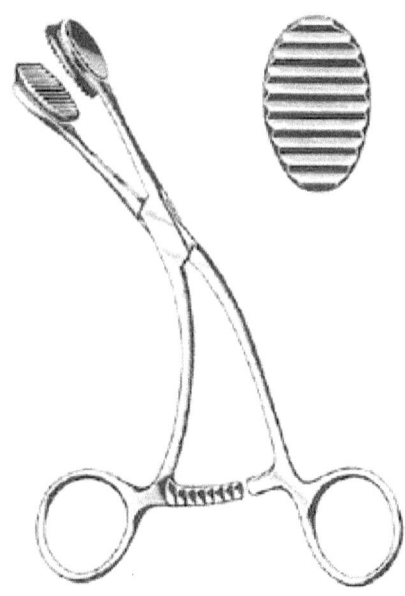

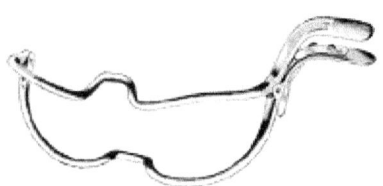

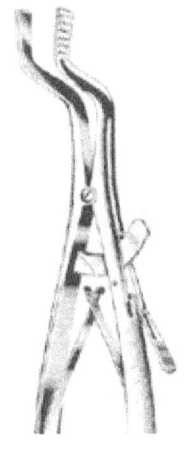

GYNAECOLOGY

Common Uses:

Vaginal speculums are used in examination of the vagina and cervix. It allows the vaginal cavity to be opened; these are also use in fertility treatments.

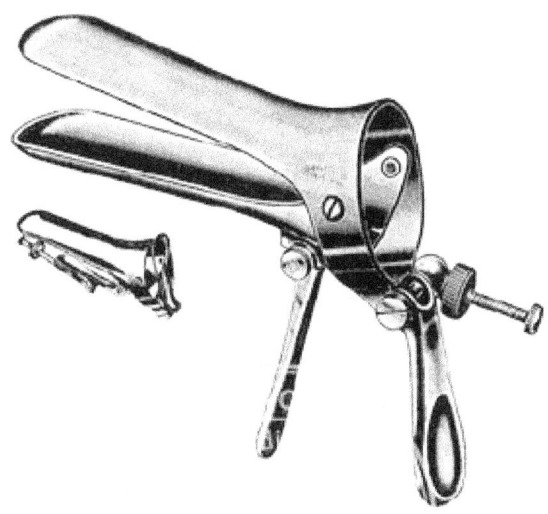

HEMOSTATIC FORCEPS

Common Uses:

Hemostatic Forceps are usually used to control bleeding, initial incision are lined with hemostats closing blood vessels awaiting ligation. Interlocking teeth keep forceps closed.

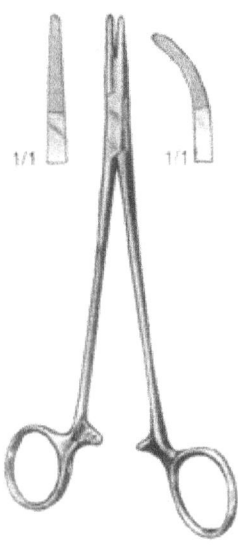

NEEDLE HOLDERS

Common Uses:

Needle holders are used to hold a suturing needle during suturing and surgical procedures.

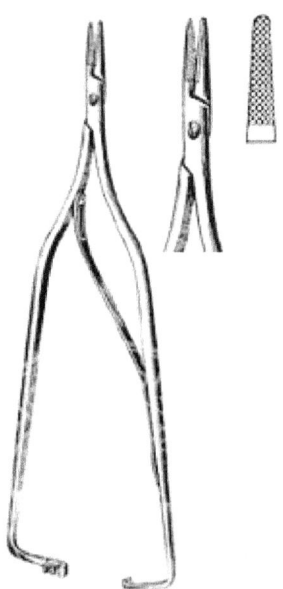

OBSTETRICAL FORCEPS

Common Uses:

Obstetrics forceps are designed to aid in the delivery of the fetus by applying traction to the fetal head.

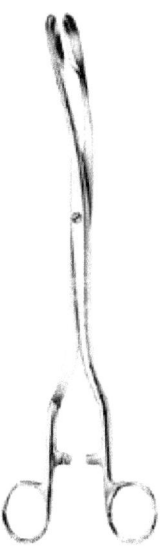

OTOLOGY

Common Uses:

Otology instruments are used in study and treatment of the Ear (hearing and vestibular sensory systems and related structures and functions) as well as its diseases, diagnosis and treatment.

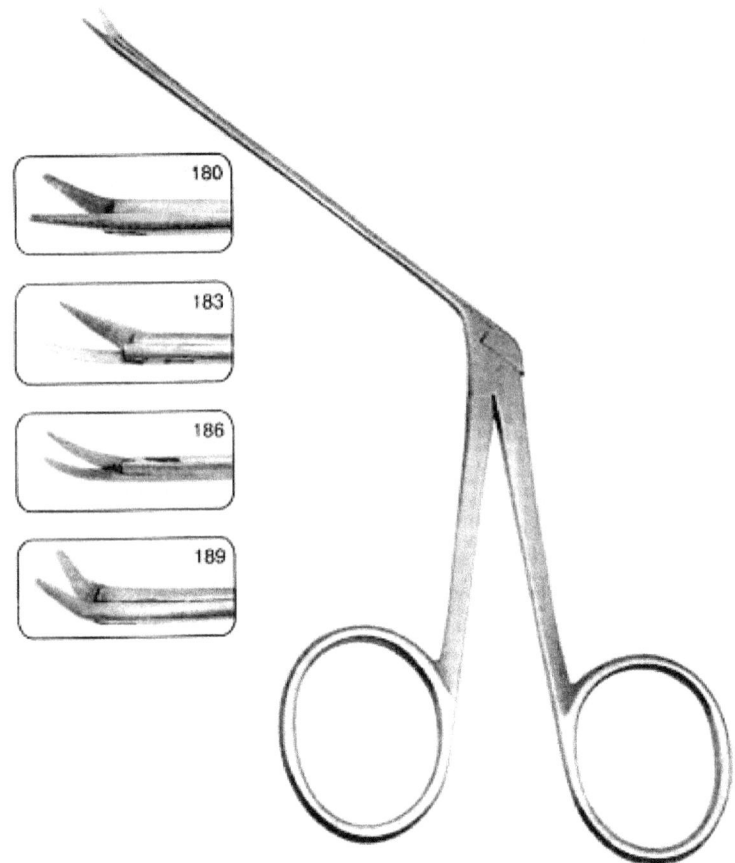

RETRACTORS

Common Uses:

Medical Tools Retractors used by surgeons to either actively separate the edges of a surgical incision or wound, or can hold back underlying organs and tissues, so that body parts under the incision may be accessed.

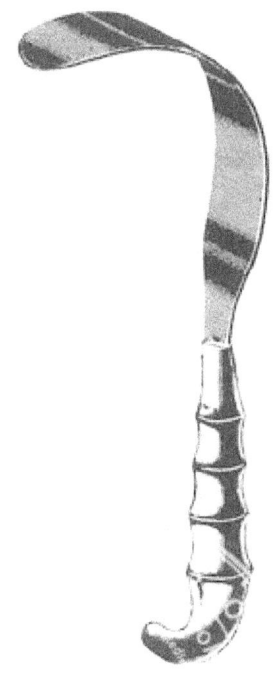

RHINOLOGY

Common Uses:

Rhinology instruments are used in Nasal and Sinus study and treatment

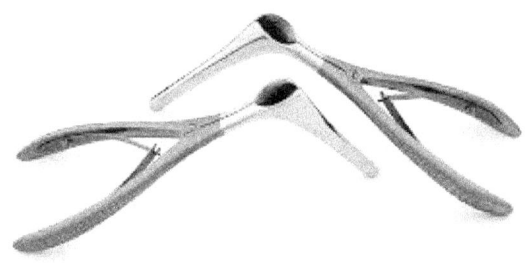

SCALPEL

Common Uses:

Scalpel handle holds a scalpel blade used for surgery and anatomical dissection.

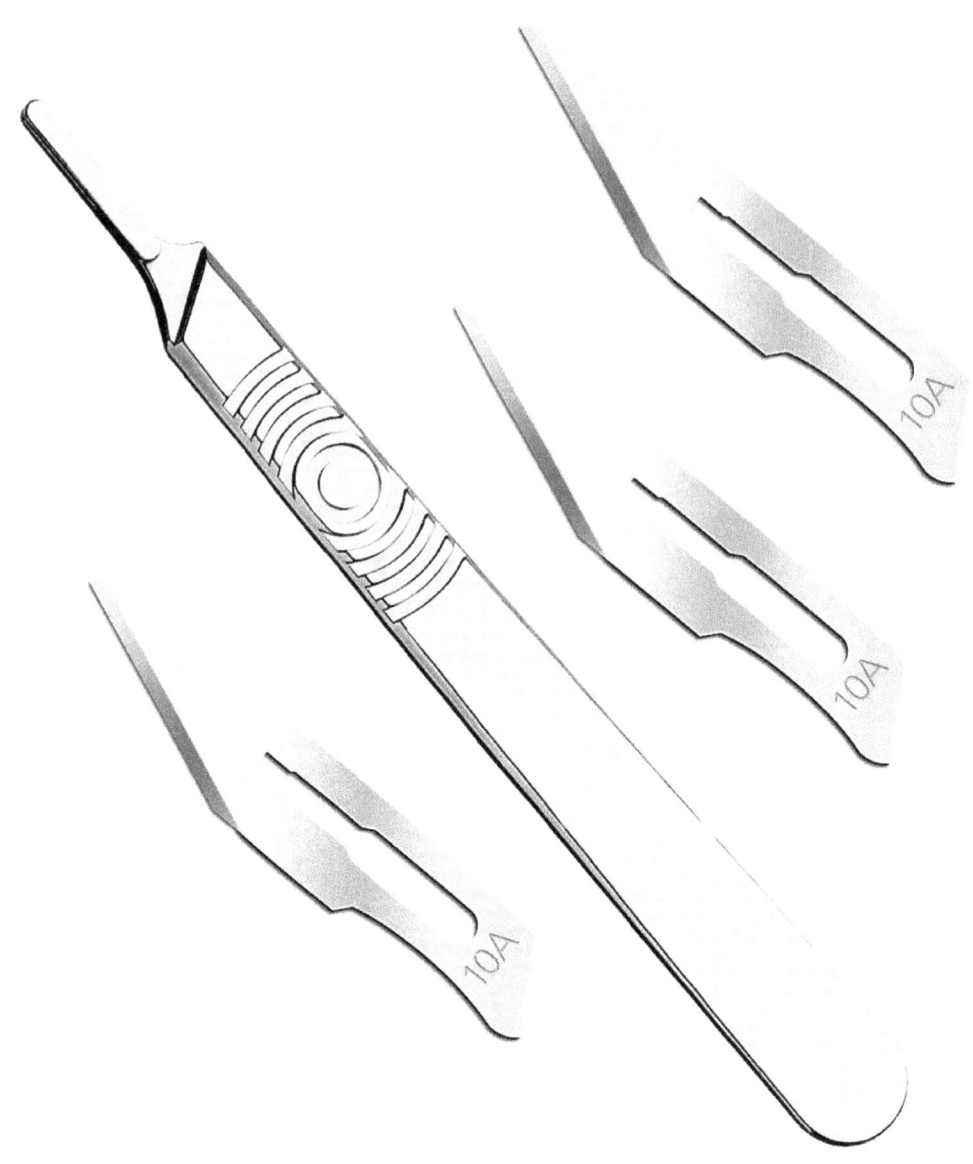

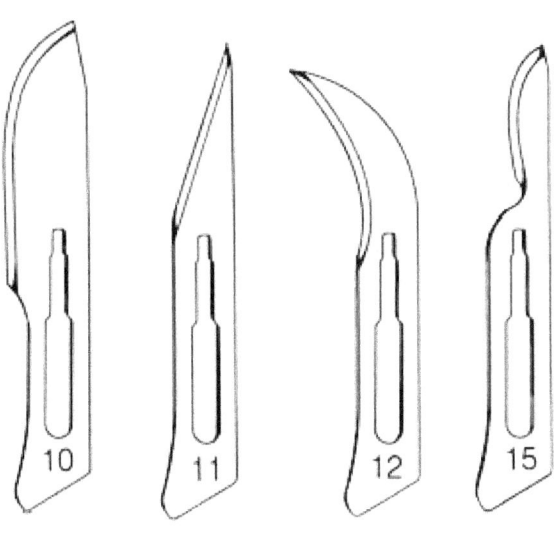
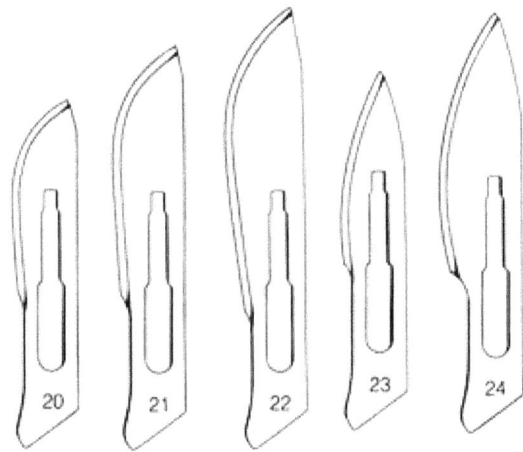
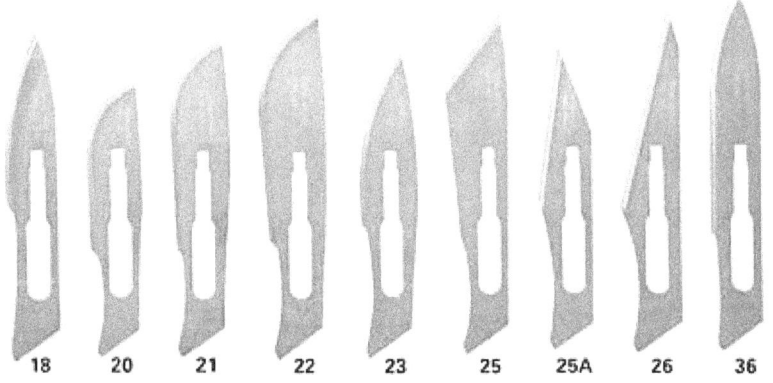

SCISSORS

Common Uses:

Medical Tools scissors are high precision cutting instruments

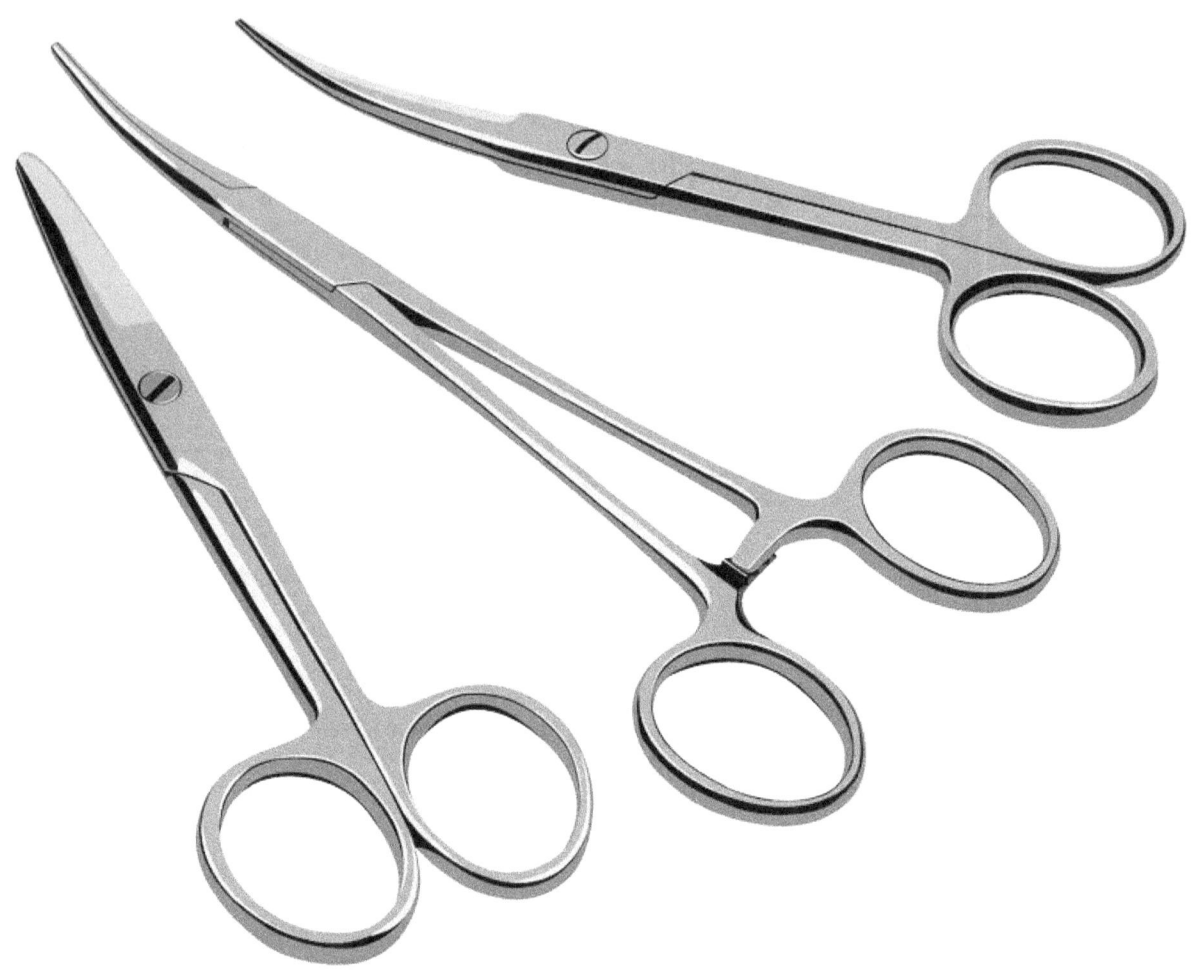

STERILIZING AIDS

Common Uses:

Sterilizing aids are used to hold instruments and help in sterilizing.

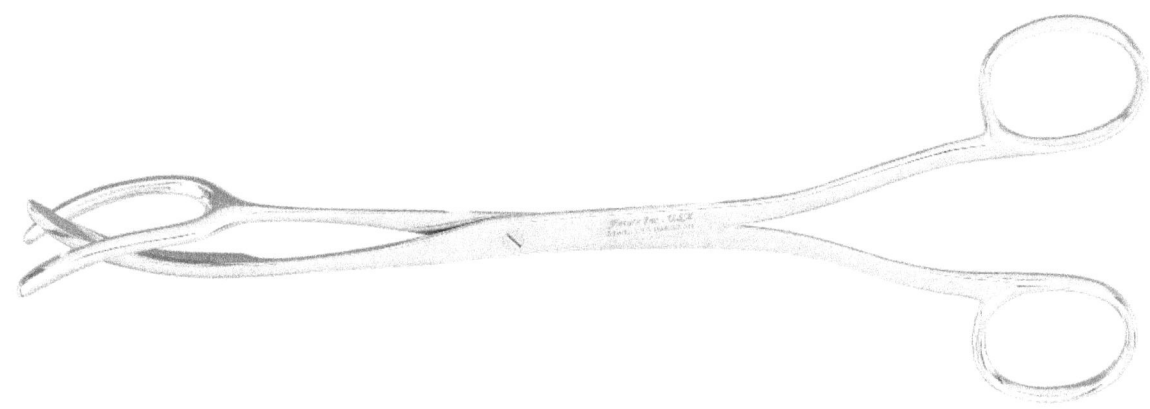

TOWEL CLAMPS

Common Uses:

A towel force is used to secure towels and surgical draping during a medical procedure.

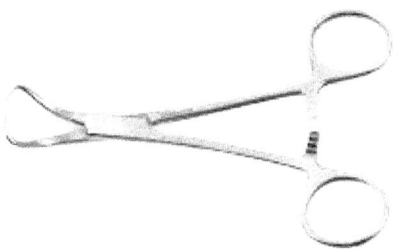

TUBING CLAMP

The tubing clamps can be used on patient drain lines, cardiac tubing and a variety of other lines that require clamping.

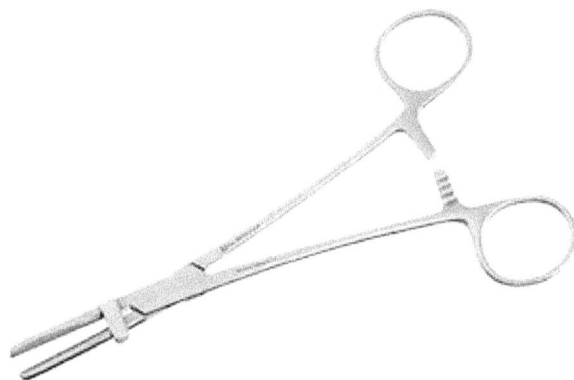

UROLOGY/KIDNEY INSTRUMENTS

Urology/Kidney Instruments are used for Urologic surgery which is the integration of surgical activities for the pelvis, the colon, urogenital, and gynecological organs. Urology Instruments are commonly used for

renal (kidney) surgery
kidney removal (nephrectomy)
surgery of the ureters, including ureter lithotomy or removal of calculus (stones) in the ureters
bladder surgery
pelvic lymph node dissection
prostatic surgery, removal of the prostate
testicular (scrotal) surgery
urethra surgery
surgery to the penis

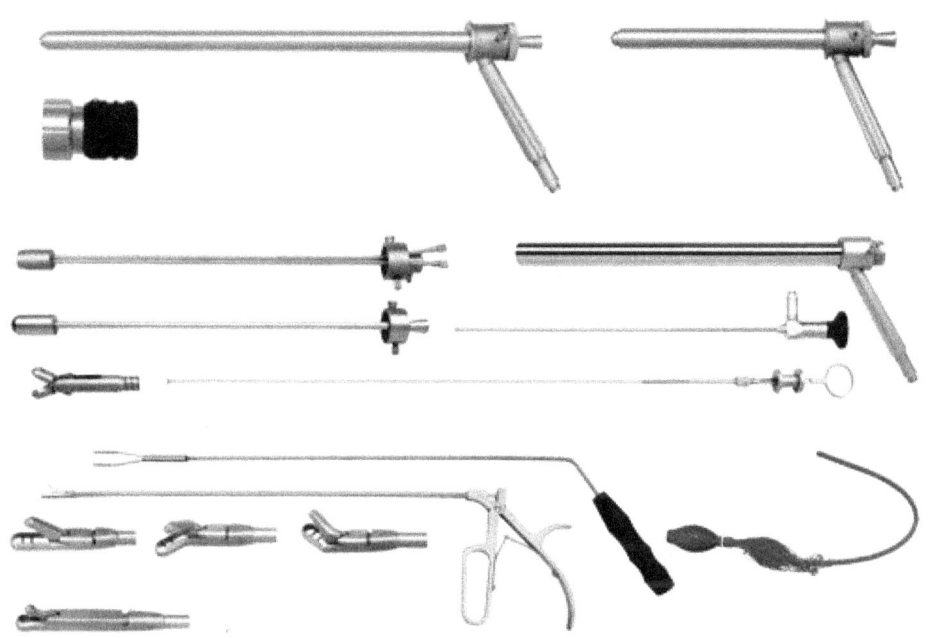

PREOPERATIVE CARE

Definition

Preoperative care is the preparation and management of a patient prior to surgery. It includes both physical and psychological preparation.

Purpose

Patients who are physically and psychologically prepared for surgery tend to have better surgical outcomes. Preoperative teaching meets the patient's need for information regarding the surgical experience, which in turn may alleviate most of his or her fears. Patients who are more knowledgeable about what to expect after surgery, and who have an opportunity to express their goals and opinions, often cope better with postoperative pain and decreased mobility. Preoperative care is extremely important prior to any invasive procedure, regardless of whether the procedure is minimally invasive or a form of major surgery.

Preoperative teaching must be individualized for each patient. Some people want as much information as possible, while others prefer only minimal information because too much knowledge may increase their anxiety. Patients have different abilities to comprehend medical procedures; some prefer printed information, while others learn more from oral presentations. It is important for the patient to ask questions during preoperative teaching sessions.

Description

Preoperative care involves many components, and may be done the day before surgery in the hospital, or during the weeks before surgery on an outpatient basis. Many surgical procedures are now performed in a day surgery setting, and the patient is never admitted to the hospital.

Physical preparation

Physical preparation may consist of a complete medical history and physical exam, including the patient's surgical and anesthesia background. The patient should inform the physician and hospital staff if he or she has ever had an adverse reaction to anesthesia (such as anaphylactic shock), or if there is a family history of malignant hyperthermia. Laboratory tests may include **complete blood count**, electrolytes, prothrombin time, activated partial thromboplastin time, and **urinalysis**. The patient will most likely have an electrocardiogram (EKG) if he or she has a history of cardiac disease, or is over 50 years of age. A **chest x ray** is done if the patient has a history of respiratory disease. Part of the preparation includes assessment for risk factors that might impair healing, such as nutritional deficiencies, steroid use, radiation or chemotherapy, drug or alcohol abuse, or metabolic diseases such as diabetes. The patient should also provide a list of all medications, vitamins, and herbal or food supplements that he or she uses. Supplements are often overlooked, but may cause adverse effects when used with general anesthetics (e.g., St. John's wort, valerian root). Some supplements can prolong bleeding time (e.g., garlic, gingko biloba).

Latex allergy has become a public health concern. Latex is found in most sterile surgical gloves, and is a common component in other medical supplies including general anesthesia masks, tubing, and multi-dose medication vials. It is estimated that 1–6% of the general population and 8–17% of health care workers have this allergy. Children with disabilities are particularly susceptible. This includes children with spina bifida, congenital urological abnormalities, cerebral palsy, and Dandy-Walker syndrome. At least 50% of children with spina bifida are latex-sensitive as a result of early, frequent surgical exposure. There is currently no cure available for latex allergy, and research has found that the allergy accounts for up to 19% of all anaphylactic reactions during surgery. The best treatment is prevention, but immediate symptomatic treatment is required if the allergic response occurs. Every patient should be assessed for a potential latex reaction. Patients with latex sensitivity should have their chart flagged with a caution label. Latex-free gloves and supplies must be used for anyone with a documented latex allergy.

Bowel clearance may be ordered if the patient is having surgery of the lower gastrointestinal tract. The patient should start the bowel preparation early the evening before surgery to prevent interrupted sleep during the night. Some patients may benefit from a sleeping pill the night before surgery.

The night before surgery, skin preparation is often ordered, which can take the form of scrubbing with a special soap (i.e., Hibiclens), or possibly hair removal from the surgical area. Shaving hair is no longer recommended because studies show that this practice may increase the chance of infection. Instead, adhesive barrier drapes can contain hair growth on the skin around the incision.

Psychological preparation

Patients are often fearful or anxious about having surgery. It is often helpful for them to express their concerns to health care workers. This can be especially beneficial for patients who are critically ill, or who are having a high-risk procedure. The family needs to be included in psychological preoperative care. Pastoral care is usually offered in the hospital. If the patient has a fear of dying during surgery, this concern should be expressed, and the surgeon notified. In some cases, the procedure may be postponed until the patient feels more secure.

Children may be especially fearful. They should be allowed to have a parent with them as much as possible, as long as the parent is not demonstrably fearful and contributing to the child's apprehension. Children should be encouraged to bring a favorite toy or blanket to the hospital on the day of surgery.

Patients and families who are prepared psychologically tend to cope better with the patient's postoperative course. Preparation leads to superior outcomes since the goals of recovery are known ahead of time, and the patient is able to manage postoperative pain more effectively.

Informed consent

The patient's or guardian's written consent for the surgery is a vital portion of preoperative care. By law, the physician who will perform the procedure must explain the risks and benefits of the surgery, along with other treatment options. However, the nurse is often the person who actually witnesses the patient's signature on the consent form. It is important that the patient understands everything he or she has been told. Sometimes, patients are asked to explain what they were told so that the health care professional can determine how much is understood.

Patients who are mentally impaired, heavily sedated, or critically ill are not considered legally able to give consent. In this situation, the next of kin (spouse, adult child, adult sibling, or person with medical **power of attorney**) may act as a surrogate and sign the consent form. Children under age 18 must have a parent or guardian sign.

Preoperative teaching

Preoperative teaching includes instruction about the preoperative period, the surgery itself, and the postoperative period.

Instruction about the preoperative period deals primarily with the arrival time, where the patient should go on the day of surgery, and how to prepare for surgery. For example, patients should be told how long they should be NPO (nothing by mouth), which medications to take prior to surgery, and the medications that should be brought with them (such as inhalers for patients with asthma).

Instruction about the surgery itself includes informing the patient about what will be done during the surgery, and how long the procedure is expected to take. The patient should be told where the incision will be. Children having surgery should be allowed to "practice" on a doll or stuffed animal. It may be helpful to demonstrate procedures on the doll prior to performing them on the child. It is also important for family members (or other concerned parties) to know where to wait during surgery, when they can expect progress information, and how long it will be before they can see the patient.

Knowledge about what to expect during the postoperative period is one of the best ways to improve the patient's outcome. Instruction about expected activities can also increase compliance and help prevent complications. This includes the opportunity for the patient to practice coughing and deep breathing exercises, use an incentive spirometer, and practice splinting the incision. Additionally, the patient should be informed about early ambulation (getting out of bed). The patient should also be taught that the respiratory interventions decrease the occurrence of pneumonia, and that early leg exercises and ambulation decrease the risk of blood clots.

Patients hospitalized postoperatively should be informed about the tubes and equipment that they will have. These may include multiple intravenous lines, drainage tubes, dressings, and monitoring devices. In addition, they may have sequential compression stockings on their legs to prevent blood clots until they start ambulating.

Pain management is the primary concern for many patients having surgery. Preoperative instruction should include information about the pain management method that they will utilize postoperatively. Patients should be encouraged to ask for or take pain medication before the pain becomes unbearable, and should be taught how to rate their discomfort on a pain scale. This instruction allows the patients, and others who may be assessing them, to evaluate the pain consistently. If they will be using a **patient-controlled analgesia** pump, instruction should take place during the preoperative period. Use of alternative methods of pain control (distraction, imagery, positioning, mindfulness meditation, music therapy) may also be presented.

Finally, the patient should understand long-term goals such as when he or she will be able to eat solid food, go home, drive a car, and return to work.

Preparation

It is important to allow adequate time for preparation prior to surgery. The patient should understand that he or she has the right to add or strike out items on the generic consent form that do not pertain to the specific surgery. For example, a patient who is about to undergo a **tonsillectomy** might choose to strike out (and initial) an item that indicates sterility might be a complication of the operation.

Normal results

The anticipated outcome of preoperative care is a patient who is informed about the surgical course, and copes with it successfully. The goal is to decrease complications and promote recovery.

INTRAOPERATIVE CARE

Definition

The term "intraoperative" refers to the time during surgery. Intraoperative care is patient care during an operation and ancillary to that operation.

Activities such as monitoring the patient's **vital signs, blood** oxygenation levels, fluid therapy, medication transfusion, anesthesia, radiography, and retrieving samples for laboratory tests, are examples of intraoperative care. Intraoperative care is provided by nurses, anesthesiologists, nurse anesthetists, surgical technicians, surgeons, and residents, all working as a team.

Purpose

The purpose of intraoperative care is to maintain patient safety and comfort during surgical procedures. Some of the goals of intraoperative care include maintaining homeostasis during the procedure, maintaining strict sterile techniques to decrease the chance of cross-infection, ensuring that the patient is secure on the operating table, and taking measures to prevent hematomas from safety strips or from positioning.

Precautions

Patients undergoing surgery most often are given some type of anesthesia. The administration of **general anesthesia** has a relaxing effect on the patient's body, which can suppress cardiovascular function or heighten cardiovascular irritability. It may also result in respiratory depression, loss of consciousness, **paralysis,** and lack of sensation. These effects, some of which are intentional for the period of the surgery, mean the patient is in a very vulnerable position. It is the responsibility of the health care team in the operating room to maintain the patient's safety and yet facilitate surgery.

In 1992, the American Association of Nurse Anesthetists (AANA) established guidelines for monitoring patients undergoing general anesthesia. The guidelines call for continuous observation of the patient by the nurse assigned to the patient. Ventilation should be assessed by continuous auscultation of breath sounds, and oxygenation should be monitored by continuous pulse oximetry. Continuous electrocardiograph (ECG) showing the patient's cardiac function should be in place, and the patient's **heart** rate and **blood pressure** should be monitored at least every five minutes. A means to monitor the patient's temperature must be available immediately for use. In case of an emergency backup personnel who are experts in **airway management,** emergency intubation, and advanced cardiac life support (ACLS) must be available. An emergency cart containing the necessary supplies and equipment must be immediately accessible. The ACLS equipment should be checked daily to ensure proper function.

Total analgesia is a goal of general anesthesia in order to facilitate surgery. This means that the patient does not have the normal "pain" sensations that warn of potential injury. The health care team must keep this in mind when they are positioning the patient for a surgical procedure.

Although it may be necessary for a patient to be positioned in an unusual way for access to a particular area during surgery, care must be taken to ensure that the patient's body is in proper alignment and that joints and muscles are not in such an unnatural position that they will be damaged if they remain in that position for a lengthy procedure. Areas of the operating table that come into contact with the patient's bony prominences must be padded to prevent skin trauma and hematomas.

During a surgical procedure many instruments, drapes, and sponges are used. Also, a multitude of care providers may be working in the operative field performing different tasks. These factors, combined with the complexity and length of some surgical procedures, may provide extensive opportunity for patient trauma from equipment malfunction or the failure of the surgical team to avoid using full weight on the sedated patient. Additionally, it is the responsibility of the nurses working in the operating room to maintain an accurate count of all sponges, instruments, and sharps that may become **foreign bodies** upon incision closure. Nurses who fail to make accurate counts can be held legally liable.

Most surgical procedures are invasive and compromise a patient's skin integrity. This increases the risk of **infection.** To decrease the risk, strict asepsis (sterile technique) must be followed at all times. It is recommended that the ventilation system in an operative area provide a minimum of fifteen exchanges of filtered air per hour. The temperature in the intraoperative area should be maintained at 68-73°F (20-23°C), and the relative humidity should be maintained at 30%-60%. Health care personnel who work in the operating room must not be permitted to work if they have open lesions on the hands or arms, eye infections, **diarrhea,** or respiratory infections. Scrub attire must be worn by all personnel entering the operating room. Fresh scrub attire must be donned daily and, if heavily soiled during one case, should be changed before the next case. Most facilities provide personnel with scrub attire that is professionally laundered. Shoe covers are required and should be changed often. Head and facial hair must be completely contained in a lint-free cap or hood. Properly fitting disposable surgical masks must be worn at all times and discarded immediately after use. Sterile gloves and sterile gowns must be worn by those working in, and in proximity to, the sterile field. Careful skin preparation with appropriate antiseptic solutions is preformed on the patient's arrival to the operating area.

Patients who have a known or suspected allergy to latex should be scheduled for surgery as the first case of the day whenever possible to avoid contact with airborne latex particles (often attached to powder granules from the gloves) that may be in the room from a previous surgery. These patients should also be identified (some facilities use special colored identification bands and colored tapes on the patient's medical record) so that all health care personnel can recognize them. Special care must be taken to limit the uses of equipment containing latex that will contact the patient's skin. This includes anesthesia masks, adhesive tape and dressings, injections drawn from multidose vials with rubber stoppers, adhesive ground plates for electrocautery or diathermy, and pad coverings on the operating table and arm extensions.

Description

Intraoperative care includes the activities performed by the health care team during surgery that ensure the patient's safety and comfort, implement the surgical procedure, monitor and maintain vital functions, and document care given. The intraoperative time period can vary greatly from less than one hour to 12 hours or more, depending on the complexity of the surgery being performed.

Preparation

Prior to surgery the patient or legal guardian must have the surgical procedure explained to them in great detail, including the expected outcomes and all possible complications, in order to give **informed consent.** The explanation should be given to the patient at a time when he or she is relaxed, but when judgment is not clouded by the use of any **pain** medication or anesthesia, which would invalidate the consent. A consent form must be signed by the patient or guardian and witnessed by a staff member as well as the surgeon performing the procedure. It is the duty of the RN admitting the patient to the surgical suite to check the patient's ID band and ensure that all records are intact and accounted for.

After consent is given the patient may be taken to a holding area where a large-bore intravenous catheter is inserted into the patient's arm for use in fluid replacement and to infuse medications during the procedure. The area of the body where the incision will be made is meticulously prepared using drapes, and a skin preparation that is antiseptic and may include the use of alcohol solutions and iodophor. Monitoring devices such as continuous ECG nodes, pulse oximetry probes, and a blood pressure cuff are usually applied prior to skin preparation. Anesthesia, also, is begun before skin prep. Surgery is then ready to begin.

Aftercare

The time after surgery is referred to as the post-operative period and includes the recovery and convalescence phases. The recovery phase is the time immediately after surgery when the effects of anesthesia are wearing off and the patient is waking up. The convalescence phase is spent either in the hospital, in an interim care facility, or at home—depending on the procedure and the preferences of the physician and patient.

Complications

Intraoperative complications are surgery related, anesthesia related, or position related. One complication occurring during the intraoperative period equipment should always be available in the event it is needed for this purpose. Another anesthesia-related complication is called "awareness under anesthesia." This occurs when the patient receives sufficient muscle relaxant (paralytic agent) to prohibit voluntary motor function but insufficient sedation and analgesia to block pain and the sense of **hearing.** Patients are aware of being "awake" because they hear the sounds and conversation in the room and, in some cases, can feel the pain associated with the skin incision and surgery. However, they cannot respond to these sensations in a waya—not even with so small a motion as blinking the eyelid—that will tell someone what they are sensing. This condition creates an exaggerated fear response that can affect hemodynamics and vital signs. Another complicating reaction may be that of malignant hyperthermia. This is a chain reaction triggered in susceptible people by commonly used general anesthetics. Signs include greatly increased body **metabolism,** muscle rigidity, and eventual hyperthermia which may exceed

110°F (43.3°C). Death may be caused by cardiac arrest, **brain** damage, internal hemorrhage, or failure of other body systems.

Complications of surgery include, but are not limited to, hypovolemic **shock** (due to blood loss during surgery), injuries from poor positioning during surgery, infection of the surgical wound, fluid and electrolyte imbalances, aspiration **pneumonia,** blood clots, and paralytic ileus (paralysis of the intestines, causing distention).

KEY TERMS

Anaphylactic reaction (anaphylaxis)— A hypersensitive reaction to an antigen resulting in life-threatening, progressive symptoms.

Anesthesia— A classification of medications that are intended to cause the loss of normal sensation.

Aseptic technique— Strict sterile procedures instilled to decrease the risk of contamination of a surgical site or open wound.

ECG— Abbreviation for electrocardiograph. Electrocardiograph is a tracing of the electrical activity of the heart obtained through electrodes placed on a person's skin in certain areas where electrical activity can be easily be detected.

Hypovolemic shock— A state of shock caused by the sudden loss of large amounts of blood.

Informed consent— Written or oral permission given by a patient or guardian for medical or surgical treatment after a complete explanation is given and any questions the patient has are answered. If consent is given orally, documentation must have two witnesses.

Intraoperative care— Care provided to a patient during surgery that is ancillary to the surgery.

Malignant hyperthermia— A chain reaction triggered in susceptible people by commonly used general anesthetics. Signs include greatly increased body metabolism, muscle rigidity, and eventual hyperthermia which may exceed 110°F (43.3°C). Death may be caused by cardiac arrest, brain damage, internal hemorrhage, or failure of other body systems.

Pulmonary function tests— Tests used to determine ventilation and perfusion capabilities of the lungs.

Pulse oximetry— A method of measuring a patient's blood oxygenation status. A measure of 100% is optimal.

Results

The results of a surgical procedure depend greatly on the procedure preformed, the skill of the surgeon, the general health of the patient preoperatively, and the ability of the patient's body to recover from the procedure. Some surgeries cure a condition (e.g., an appendectomy for an inflamed appendix). Others are only one step in a long process to cure a disease or repair an injury (e.g., discectomy for a patient suffering from back pain). Still others are performed as palliative measures rather than as a cure. An example of palliative surgery would be the removal of a metastatic abdominal tumor to relieve abdominal pressure. In this example removing the abdominal tumor is not going to cure the **cancer** that exists in other parts of the patient's body; it is simply going to relieve the discomfort caused by the abdominal mass.

POSTOPERATIVE CARE

Definition

Postoperative care is the management of a patient after surgery. This includes care given during the immediate postoperative period, both in the **operating room** and postanesthesia care unit (PACU), as well as during the days following surgery.

Purpose

The goal of postoperative care is to prevent complications such as infection, to promote healing of the surgical incision, and to return the patient to a state of health.

Description

Postoperative care involves assessment, diagnosis, planning, intervention, and outcome evaluation. The extent of postoperative care required depends on the individual's pre-surgical health status, type of surgery, and whether the surgery was performed in a day-surgery setting or in the hospital. Patients who have procedures done in a day-surgery center usually require only a few hours of care by health care professionals before they are discharged to go home. If postanesthesia or postoperative complications occur within these hours, the patient must be admitted to the hospital. Patients who are admitted to the hospital may require days or weeks of postoperative care by hospital staff before they are discharged.

Postanesthesia care unit (PACU)

The patient is transferred to the PACU after the surgical procedure, anesthesia reversal, and extubation (if it was necessary). The amount of time the patient spends in the PACU depends on the length of surgery, type of surgery, status of regional anesthesia (e.g., spinal anesthesia), and the patient's level of consciousness. Rather than being sent to the PACU, some patients may be transferred directly to the critical care unit. For example, patients who have had coronary artery bypass grafting are sent directly to the critical care unit.

In the PACU, the anesthesiologist or the nurse anesthetist reports on the patient's condition, type of surgery performed, type of anesthesia given, estimated blood loss, and total input of fluids and output of urine during surgery. The PACU nurse should also be made aware of any complications during surgery, including variations in hemodynamic (blood circulation) stability.

Assessment of the patient's airway patency (openness of the airway), **vital signs**, and level of consciousness are the first priorities upon admission to the PACU. The following is a list of other assessment categories:

surgical site (intact dressings with no signs of overt bleeding)
patency (proper opening) of drainage tubes/drains
body temperature (hypothermia/hyperthermia)
patency/rate of intravenous (IV) fluids

circulation/sensation in extremities after vascular or orthopedic surgery
level of sensation after regional anesthesia
pain status
nausea/vomiting

The patient is discharged from the PACU when he or she meets established criteria for discharge, as determined by a scale. One example is the Aldrete scale, which scores the patient's mobility, respiratory status, circulation, consciousness, and pulse oximetry. Depending on the type of surgery and the patient's condition, the patient may be admitted to either a general surgical floor or the **intensive care unit**. Since the patient may still be sedated from anesthesia, safety is a primary goal. The patient's call light should be in the hand and side rails up. Patients in a day surgery setting are either discharged from the PACU to the unit, or are directly discharged home after they have urinated, gotten out of bed, and tolerated a small amount of oral intake.

After the hospitalized patient transfers from the PACU, the nurse taking over his or her care should assess the patient again, using the same previously mentioned categories. If the patient reports "hearing" or feeling pain during surgery (under anesthesia) the observation should not be discounted. The anesthesiologist or nurse anesthetist should discuss the possibility of an episode of awareness under anesthesia with the patient. Vital signs, respiratory status, pain status, the incision, and any drainage tubes should be monitored every one to two hours for at least the first eight hours. Body temperature must be monitored, since patients are often hypothermic after surgery, and may need a warming blanket or warmed IV fluids. Respiratory status should be assessed frequently, including assessment of lung sounds (auscultation) and chest excursion, and presence of an adequate cough. Fluid intake and urine output should be monitored every one to two hours. If the patient does not have a urinary catheter, the bladder should be assessed for distension, and the patient monitored for inability to urinate. The physician should be notified if the patient has not urinated six to eight hours after surgery. If the patient had a vascular or neurological procedure performed, circulatory status or neurological status should be assessed as ordered by the surgeon, usually every one to two hours. The patient may require medication for nausea or vomiting, as well as pain.

Patients with a **patient-controlled analgesia** pump may need to be reminded how to use it. If the patient is too sedated immediately after the surgery, the nurse may push the button to deliver pain medication. The patient should be asked to rate his or her pain level on a pain scale in order to determine his or her acceptable level of pain. Controlling pain is crucial so that the patient may perform coughing, deep breathing exercises, and may be able to turn in bed, sit up, and, eventually, walk.

Effective preoperative teaching has a positive impact on the first 24 hours after surgery. If patients understand that they must perform respiratory exercises to prevent pneumonia; and that movement is imperative for preventing blood clots, encouraging circulation to the extremities, and keeping the lungs clear; they will be much more likely to perform these tasks. Understanding the need for movement and respiratory exercises also underscores the importance of keeping pain under control. Respiratory exercises (coughing, deep breathing, and incentive spirometry) should be done every two hours. The patient should be turned every two hours, and should at least be sitting on the edge of the bed by eight hours after surgery, unless contraindicated (e.g., after **hip replacement**). Patients who are not able to sit up in bed due to their surgery will have sequential compression devices on their legs until they are able to move about. These are stockings that inflate with air in order to simulate the effect of walking on the calf muscles, and return blood to the heart. The patient should be encouraged to splint any chest and abdominal incisions with a pillow to decrease the pain caused by coughing and moving. Patients should be kept NPO (nothing by mouth) if ordered by the surgeon, at least until their cough and gag reflexes have returned. Patients often have a dry mouth following surgery, which can be relieved with oral sponges dipped in ice water or lemon ginger mouth swabs.

Patients who are discharged home after a day surgery procedure are given prescriptions for their pain medications, and are responsible for their own pain control and respiratory exercises. Their families (or caregivers) should be included in preoperative teaching so that they can assist the patient at home. The patient should be reminded to call his or her physician if any complications or uncontrolled pain arise. These patients are often managed at home on a follow-up basis by a hospital-connected visiting nurse or **home care** service.

After 24 hours

After the initial 24 hours, vital signs can be monitored every four to eight hours if the patient is stable. The incision and dressing should be monitored for the amount of drainage and signs of infection. The surgeon may order a dressing change during the first postoperative day; this should be done using sterile technique. For home-care patients this technique must be emphasized.

The hospitalized patient should be sitting up in a chair at the bedside and ambulating with assistance by this time. Respiratory exercises are still be performed every two hours, and incentive spirometry values should improve. Bowel sounds are monitored, and the patient's diet gradually increased as tolerated, depending on the type of surgery and the physician's orders.

The patient should be monitored for any evidence of potential complications, such as leg edema, redness, and pain (deep vein thrombosis), shortness of breath (pulmonary embolism), dehiscence (separation) of the incision, or ileus (intestinal obstruction). The surgeon should be notified immediately if any of these occur. If dehiscence occurs, sterile saline-soaked dressing packs should be placed on the wound.

Preparation

Patients receive a great deal of information on postoperative care. They may be offered pain medication in preparation for any procedure that is likely to cause discomfort. Patients may receive educational materials such as handouts and video tapes, so that they will have a clear understanding of what to expect postoperatively.

Aftercare

Aftercare includes ensuring that patients are comfortable, either in bed or chair, and that they have their call lights accessible. After dressing changes, blood-soaked dressings should be properly disposed of in a bio-hazard container. Pain medication should be offered before any procedure that might cause discomfort. Patients should be given the opportunity to ask questions. In some cases, they may ask the nurse to demonstrate certain techniques so that they can perform them properly once they return home.

Normal results

The goal of postoperative care is to ensure that patients have good outcomes after surgical procedures. A good outcome includes recovery without complications and adequate **pain management**. Another objective of postoperative care is to assist patients in taking responsibility for regaining optimum health.

NEUROLOGY

Neurology is a branch of medicine dealing with disorders of the nervous system. Neurology deals with the diagnosis and treatment of all categories of conditions and disease involving the central and peripheral systems (and its subdivisions, the autonomic nervous system and the somatic nervous system); including their coverings, blood vessels, and all effector tissue, such as muscle. Neurological practice relies heavily on the field of neuroscience, which is the scientific study of the nervous system.

A neurological examination assesses motor and sensory skills, the functioning of one or more cranial nerves, hearing and speech, vision, coordination and balance, mental status, and changes in mood or behavior, among other abilities.

Items including a tuning fork, flashlight, reflex hammer, ophthalmoscope, and needles are used to help diagnose brain tumors, infections such as encephalitis and meningitis, and diseases such as Parkinson's disease, Huntington's disease, amyotrophic lateral sclerosis (ALS), and epilepsy. Some tests require the services of a specialist to perform and analyze results.

X-rays of the patient's chest and skull are often taken as part of a neurological work-up. X-rays can be used to view any part of the body, such as a joint or major organ system. In a conventional x-ray, also called a radiograph, a technician passes a concentrated burst of low-dose ionized radiation through the body and onto a photographic plate.

Since calcium in bones absorbs x-rays more easily than soft tissue or muscle, the bony structure appears white on the film. Any vertebral misalignment or fractures can be seen within minutes. Tissue masses such as injured ligaments or a bulging disc are not visible on conventional x-rays. This fast, noninvasive, painless procedure is usually performed in a doctor's office or at a clinic.

Fluoroscopy is a type of x-ray that uses a continuous or pulsed beam of low-dose radiation to produce continuous images of a body part in motion. The fluoroscope (x-ray tube) is focused on the area of interest and pictures are either videotaped or sent to a monitor for viewing. A contrast medium may be used to highlight the images. Fluoroscopy can be used to evaluate the flow of blood through arteries.

TESTS

Laboratory screening tests of blood, urine, or other substances are used to help diagnose disease, better understand the disease process, and monitor levels of therapeutic drugs. Certain tests, ordered by the physician as part of a regular check-up, provide general information, while others are used to identify specific health concerns.

For example, blood and blood product tests can detect brain and/or spinal cord infection, bone marrow disease, hemorrhage, blood vessel damage, toxins that affect the nervous system, and the presence of antibodies that signal the presence of an autoimmune disease. Blood tests are also used to monitor levels of therapeutic drugs used to treat epilepsy and other neurological disorders. Genetic testing of DNA extracted from white cells in the blood can help diagnose Huntington's disease and other congenital diseases.

Analysis of the fluid that surrounds the brain and spinal cord can detect meningitis, acute and chronic inflammation, rare infections, and some cases of multiple sclerosis. Chemical and metabolic testing of the blood can indicate protein disorders, some forms of muscular dystrophy and other muscle disorders, and diabetes. Urinalysis can reveal abnormal substances in the urine or the presence or absence of certain proteins that cause diseases including the mucopolysaccharidoses.

Genetic testing or counseling can help parents who have a family history of a neurological disease determine if they are carrying one of the known genes that cause the disorder or find out if their child is affected. Genetic testing can identify many neurological disorders, including spina bifida, in utero (while the child is inside the mother's womb).

Genetic tests include the following:

-*Amniocentesis*, usually done at 14-16 weeks of pregnancy, tests a sample of the amniotic fluid in the womb for genetic defects (the fluid and the fetus have the same DNA). Under local anesthesia, a thin needle is inserted through the woman's abdomen and into the womb. About 20 milliliters of fluid (roughly 4 teaspoons) is withdrawn and sent to a lab for evaluation. Test results often take 1-2 weeks.

-*Chorionic villus sampling*, or CVS, is performed by removing and testing a very small sample of the placenta during early pregnancy. The sample, which contains the same DNA as the fetus, is removed by catheter or fine needle inserted through the cervix or by a fine needle inserted through the abdomen. It is tested for genetic abnormalities and results are usually available within 2 weeks. CVS should not be performed after the tenth week of pregnancy.

-*Uterine ultrasound* is performed using a surface probe with gel. This noninvasive test can suggest the diagnosis of conditions such as chromosomal disorders

Specific tests in a neurological examination include:

-Examination of posture
-Decerebrate
-Decorticat
-Hemiparetic
-Abnormal movements
-Seizure
-Fasciculations
-Cerebellar testing
-Dysmetria
-Finger-to-nose test

-Ankle-over-tibia test
-Dysdiadochokinesis
-Rapid pronation-supination
-Ataxia
-Assessment of gait
-Nystagmus
-Intension tremor
-Staccato speech
-Tone
-Spasticity
-Pronator drift
-Rigidity
-Cogwheeling (abnormal tone suggestive of Parkinson's disease)
-Gegenhalten – is resistance to passive change, where the strength of antagonist muscles increases with increasing examiner force. More common in dementia.
-Romberg test to examine proprioception or cerebellar function
-Resting tremors
-Sensory
-Light touch
-Pain
-Temperature
-Vibration
-Position sense
-Graphesthesia
-Stereognosis, and
-Two-point discrimination (for discriminative sense)
-Extinction

DISORDERS

A **neurological disorder** is any disorder of the nervous system. Structural, biochemical or electrical abnormalities in the brain, spinal cord or other nerves can result in a range of symptoms. Examples of symptoms include paralysis, muscle weakness, poor coordination, loss of sensation, seizures, confusion, pain and altered levels of consciousness. There are many recognized neurological disorders, some relatively common, but many rare. They may be assessed by neurological examination, and studied and treated within the specialties of neurology and clinical neuropsychology.

Interventions for neurological disorders include preventative measures, lifestyle changes, neurorehabilitation, pain management, medication, or operations performed by neurosurgeons. The World Health Organization estimated in 2006 that neurological disorders and their direct consequences affect as many as one billion people worldwide, and identified health inequalities and discrimination as major factors contributing to the associated disability and suffering.

CAUSES

Although the brain and spinal cord are surrounded by tough membranes, enclosed in the bones of the skull and spinal vertebrae, and chemically isolated by the so-called blood-brain barrier, they are very susceptible if compromised. Nerves tend to lie deep under the skin but can still become exposed to damage. Individual neurons, and the neural networks and nerves into which they form, are susceptible to electrochemical and structural disruption.

The specific causes of neurological problems vary, but can include genetic disorders, congenital abnormalities or disorders, infections, lifestyle or environmental health problems including malnutrition, and brain injury, spinal cord injury or nerve injury. The problem may start in another body system that interacts with the nervous system. For example, cerebrovascular disorders involve brain injury due to problems with the blood vessels supplying the brain; autoimmune disorders involve damage caused by the body's own immune system; dieseases such as neimann-pick disease can lead to neurological deterioration.

In a substantial minority of cases of neurological symptoms, no neural cause can be identified using current testing procedures, and such "idiopathic" conditions can invite different theories about what is occurring.

CLASSIFICATION

Neurological disorders can be categorized according to the primary location affected, the primary type of dysfunction involved, or the primary type of cause. The broadest division is between central nervous systems disorders and peripheral nervous system disorders. The Merck manual lists brain, spinal cord and nerve disorders in the following overlapping categories.

Brain:

Brain damage according to central lobe

-Frontal lobe damage

-Parietal lobe damage

-Temporal Lobe damage

-Occipital lobe damage

Brain dysfunction according to type:

-Aphasia (language)

-Dysgraphia (writing)

-Dysarthria (speech)

<u>Apraxia</u> (patterns or sequences of movements)

-Agnosia (identifying things or people)

-Amnesia (memory)

Spinal cord disorders

-Peripheral nervous system disorders

-Cranial nerve disorder

-Autonomic nervous system disorders

-Seizure disorders

Movement disorders of the central and peripheral nervous system such as:

-Parkinson's disease

-Essential tremor

-Amyotrophic disorder

-Tourette's syndrome

-Multiple sclerosis

Sleep disorders

Neuropsychiatric illnesses (diseases and/or disorders with psychiatric features associated with known nervous system injury, underdevelopment, biochemical, anatomical, or electrical malfunction, and/or disease pathology

Many of the diseases and disorders listed above have neurosurgical treatments available

Others Include:

-Dementia

-Vertigo

-Head Injury

-Coma

-Stroke

-Tumors

MICROBIOLOGY

Microbiology is the study of microscopic organisms (microbes), which are defined as any living organism that is either a single cell (unicellular), a cell cluster, or has no cells at all (acellular). This includes eukaryotes, such as fungi and protists, and prokaryotes. Viruses and prions, though not strictly classed as living organisms, are also studied.

Microbiology typically includes the study of the immune system, or immunology. Generally, immune systems interact with pathogenic microbes; these two disciplines often intersect which is why many colleges offer a paired degree such as "Microbiology and Immunology"

Microbiology is a broad term which includes virology, mycology, parasitology, bacteriology, immunology, and other branches. A microbiologist is a specialist in microbiology and these related topics. Microbiological procedures usually must be aseptic and use a variety of tools such as light microscopes with a combination of stains and dyes. As microbes are absolutely required for most facets of human life (including the air we breathe and the food we eat) and are potential causes of many human diseases, microbiology is paramount for human society.

Research in the microbiology field is expanding, and in the coming years, we should see the demand for microbiologists in the workforce increase. It is estimated that only about one percent of the microorganisms present in a given environmental sample are culturable and the number of bacterial cells and species on Earth is still not possible to be determined. Recent estimates indicate that this number might be extremely high at five to the power of thirty. Although microbes were directly observed over three hundred years ago, the precise determination, quantitation, and description of its functions is far from complete, given the overwhelming diversity detected by genetic and culture-independent means.

What Are Microbes?

A microbe or microorganism is a microscopic organism that comprises either a single cell (unicellular), cell clusters, or multicellular relatively complex organisms. The study of microorganisms is called microbiology, a subject that began with Anton van Leeuwenhoek's discovery of microorganisms in 1675, using a microscope of his own design.

Microorganisms are very diverse; they include bacteria, fungi, algae, and protozoa; microscopic plants (green algae); and animals such as rotifers and planarians. Some microbiologists also include viruses, but others consider these as nonliving. Most microorganisms are unicellular, but this is not universal, since some multicellular organisms are microscopic. Some unicellular protists and bacteria, like *Thiomargarita namibiensis*, are macroscopic and visible to the naked eye.

Microorganisms live in all parts of the biosphere where there is liquid water, including soil, hot springs, on the ocean floor, high in the atmosphere, and deep inside rocks within the Earth's crust. Most importantly, these organisms are vital to humans and the environment, as they participate in the Earth's element cycles such as the carbon cycle and the nitrogen cycle. Microorganisms also fulfill other vital roles in virtually all ecosystems, such as recycling other organisms' dead remains and waste products through decomposition. Microbes also have an important place in most higher-order multicellular organisms as symbionts, and they are also exploited by people inbiotechnology, both in traditional food and beverage preparation, and in modern technologies based on genetic engineering. However, pathogenic microbes are harmful, since they invade and grow within other organisms, causing diseases that kill humans, animals, and plants.

The Pathogenic Ecology of Microbes

Although many microorganisms are beneficial, many others are the cause of infectious diseases. The organisms involved include pathogenic bacteria, which are the cause of diseases such as plague, tuberculosis and anthrax. Biofilms, microbial communities that are very difficult to destroy, are considered responsible for diseases such as bacterial infections in patients with cystic fibrosis, Legionnaires' disease, and otitis media. They produce dental plaque; colonize catheters, prostheses, transcutaneous, and orthopedic devices; and infect contact lenses, open wounds, and burned tissue.

Biofilms also produce foodborne diseases because they colonize the surfaces of food and food-processing equipment. Biofilms are a large threat because they are resistant to most of the methods used to control microbial growth. Moreover, the excessive use of antibiotics has resulted in a major global problem since resistant forms of bacteria have been selected over time. A very dangerous strain, methicillin-resistant *Staphylococcus aureus* (MRSA), has wreaked havoc recently.

In addition, protozoans are known to cause diseases such as malaria, sleeping sickness and toxoplasmosis, while fungi can cause diseases such as ringworm, candidiasis or histoplasmosis. Other diseases such as influenza, yellow fever or AIDS are caused by viruses.

Moreover, foodborne diseases result from the consumption of contaminated food, pathogenic bacteria, viruses, or parasites that contaminate food. Hygiene is the avoidance of infection or food spoiling by eliminating microorganisms from the surroundings. As microorganisms, in particular bacteria, are found virtually everywhere, the levels of harmful microorganisms can be reduced to acceptable levels with proper hygiene techniques. However, in some cases, it is required that an object or substance be completely sterile, i.e. devoid of all living entities and viruses. A good example of this is a hypodermic needle.

KEY POINTS

While most microbes are unicellular, some multicellular animals and plants are microscopic and broadly defined as microbes.

Microbes serve many functions in almost any ecosystem on the Earth, including decomposition and nitrogen fixation.

Many microbes are pathogens or parasitic organisms that can harm humans.

TERMS

symbiote
An organism in a partnership with another such that each profits from their being together.

pathogenic
Able to cause harmful disease.

ecosystem
The interconnectedness of plants, animals, and microbes with each other and their environment.

Types of Microorganisms

Microorganisms or microbes are microscopic organisms that exist as unicellular, multicellular, or cell clusters. Microorganisms are widespread in nature and are beneficial to life, but some can cause serious harm. They can be divided into six major types: bacteria, archaea, fungi, protozoa, algae, and viruses.

Bacteria

Bacteria are unicellular organisms. The cells are described as prokaryotic because they lack a nucleus. They exist in four major shapes: bacillus (rod shape), coccus (spherical shape), spirilla (spiral shape), and vibrio (curved shape). Most bacteria divide by binary fission; and they may possess flagella for motility. The difference in their cell wall structure is a major feature used in classifying these organisms.

According to the way their cell wall structure stains, bacteria can be classified as either Gram-positive or gram-negative when using the Gram staining. Bacteria can be further divided based on their response to gaseous oxygen into the following groups: aerobic (living in the presence of oxygen), anaerobic (living without oxygen), and facultative anaerobes (can live in both environments).

According to the way they obtain energy, bacteria are classified as heterotrophs or autotrophs. Autotrophs make their own food by using the energy of sunlight or chemical reactions, in which case they are called chemoautotrophs. Heterotrophs obtain their energy by consuming other organisms. Bacteria that use decaying life forms as a source of energy are called saprophytes.

Archaea

Archaea or Archaebacteria differ from true bacteria in their cell wall structure and lack peptidoglycans. They are prokaryotic cells with avidity to extreme environmental conditions. Based on their habitat, all Archaeans can be divided into the following groups: methanogens (methane-producing organisms), halophiles (archaeans that live in salty environments), thermophiles (archaeans that live at extremely hot temperatures), and psychrophiles (cold-temperature Archaeans). Archaeans use different energy sources like hydrogen gas, carbon dioxide, and sulphur. Some of them use sunlight to make energy, but not the same way plants do. They absorb sunlight using their membrane pigment, bacteriorhodopsin. This reacts with light, leading to the formation of the energy molecule adenosine triphosphate (ATP).

Fungi

Fungi (mushroom, molds, and yeasts) are eukaryotic cells (with a true nucleus). Most fungi are multicellular and their cell wall is composed of chitin. They obtain nutrients by absorbing organic material from their environment (decomposers), through symbiotic relationships with plants (symbionts), or harmful relationships with a host (parasites). They form characteristic filamentous tubes called hyphae that help absorb material. The collection of hyphae is called mycelium. Fungi reproduce by releasing spores.

Protozoa

Protozoa are unicellular aerobic eukaryotes. They have a nucleus, complex organelles, and obtain nourishment by absorption or ingestion through specialized structures. They make up the largest group of organisms in the world in terms of numbers, biomass, and diversity. Their cell walls are made up of cellulose. Protozoa have been traditionally divided based on their mode of locomotion: flagellates produce their own food and use their whip-like structure to propel forward, ciliates have tiny hair that beat to produce movement, amoeboids have false feet or pseudopodia used for feeding and locomotion, and sporozoans are non-motile. They also have different means of nutrition, which groups them as autotrophs or heterotrophs.

Algae

Algae, also called cyanobacteria or blue-green algae, are unicellular or multicellular eukaryotes that obtain nourishment by photosynthesis. They live in water, damp soil, and rocks and produce oxygen and carbohydrates used by other organisms. It is believed that cyanobacteria are the origins of green land plants.

Viruses

Viruses are noncellular entities that consist of a nucleic acid core (DNA or RNA) surrounded by a protein coat. Although viruses are classified as microorganisms, they are not considered living organisms. Viruses cannot reproduce outside a host cell and cannot metabolize on their own. Viruses often infest prokaryotic and eukaryotic cells causing diseases.

Multicellular Animal Parasites

A group of eukaryotic organisms consisting of the flatworms and roundworms, which are collectively referred to as the helminths. Although they are not microorganisms by definition, since they are large enough to be easily seen with the naked eye, they live a part of their life cycle in microscopic form. Since the parasitic helminths are of clinical importance, they are often discussed along with the other groups of microbes.

KEY POINTS

Microorganisms are divided into seven types: bacteria, archaea, protozoa, algae, fungi, viruses, and multicellular animal parasites (helminths).

Each type has a characteristic cellular composition, morphology, mean of locomotion, and reproduction.

Microorganisms are beneficial in producing oxygen, decomposing organic material, providing nutrients for plants, and maintaining human health, but some can be pathogenic and cause diseases in plants and humans.

TERMS

peptidoglycan
A polymer of glycan and peptides found in bacterial cell walls.

Gram stain
A method of differentiating bacterial species into two large groups (Gram-positive and Gram-negative).

CLASSIFICATION OF MICROORGANISMS

Life on Earth is famous for its diversity. Throughout the world we can find many millions of different forms of life. Biologic classification helps identify each form according to common properties (similarities) using a set of rules and an estimate as to how closely related it is to a common ancestor (evolutionary relationship) in a way to create an order. By learning to recognize certain patterns and classify them into specific groups, biologists are better able to understand the relationships that exist among a variety of living forms that inhabit the planet. The first, largest, and most inclusive group under which organisms are classified is called a domain and has three subgroups: bacteria, archae, and eukarya. This first group defines whether an organism is a prokaryote or a eukaryote. The domain was proposed by the microbiologist and physicist Carl Woese in 1978 and is based on identifying similarities in ribosomal RNA sequences of microorganisms.

The second largest group is called a kingdom. Five major kingdoms have been described and include prokaryota (e.g. archae and bacteria), protoctista (e.g. protozoa and algae), fungi, plantae, and animalia. A kingdom is further split into phylum or division, class, order, family, genus, and species, which is the smallest group

The science of classifying organisms is called <u>taxonomy</u> and the groups making up the classification hierarchy are called taxa. Taxonomy consists of classifying new organisms or reclassifying existing ones. Microorganisms are scientifically recognized using a binomial nomenclature using two words that refer to the genus and the species. The names assigned to microorganisms are in Latin. The first letter of the genus name is always capitalized. Classification of microorganisms has been largely aided by studies of fossils and recently by <u>DNA</u> <u>sequencing</u>. Methods of classifications are constantly changing. The most widely employed methods for classifying <u>microbes</u> are morphological characteristics, differential staining, biochemical testing, <u>DNA fingerprinting</u> or DNA base composition, <u>polymerase</u> <u>chain</u> <u>reaction</u>, and DNA chips.

KEY POINTS

The classification system is constantly changing with the advancement of technology.
The most recent classification system includes five kingdoms that are further split into phylum, class, order, family, genus, and species.
Microorganisms are assigned a scientific name using binomial nomenclature.

TERM

DNA fingerprinting
A method of isolating and mapping sequences of a cell's DNA to identify it.

APPLIED MICROBIOLOGY

Microbiology is the study of microbes, which affect almost every aspect of life on the earth. In addition, there are huge commercial and medicinal benefits in understanding microbes. The application of this understanding is known as applied microbiology. There are many different types of applied microbiology which can be briefly defined as follows:

Medical Microbiology

Medical microbiology is the study of the pathogenic microbes and the role of microbes in human illness. This includes the study of microbial pathogenesis and epidemiology and is related to the study of disease pathology and immunology.

Pharmaceutical Microbiology

The study of microorganisms that are related to the production of antibiotics, enzymes, vitamins, vaccines, and other pharmaceutical products. Pharmaceutical microbiology also studies the causes of pharmaceutical contamination and spoil.

Industrial Microbiology

The exploitation of microbes for use in industrial processes. Examples include industrial fermentation and waste-water treatment. Closely linked to the biotechnology industry. This field also includes brewing, an important application of microbiology.

Microbial Biotechnology

The manipulation of microorganisms at the genetic and molecular level to generate useful products.

Food Microbiology and Dairy Microbiology

The study of microorganisms causing food spoilage and food-borne illness. Microorganisms can produce foods, for example by fermentation .

Agricultural Microbiology

The study of agriculturally relevant microorganisms. This field can be further classified into the following subfields:

-Plant microbiology and plant pathology - The study of the interactions between microorganisms and plants and plant pathogens.

-Soil microbiology - The study of those microorganisms that are found in soil.

-Veterinary microbiology - The study of the role in microbes in veterinary medicine or animal taxonomy.

-Environmental microbiology - The study of the function and diversity of microbes in their natural environments. This involves the characterization of key bacterial habitats such as the rhizosphere and phyllosphere, soil and groundwater ecosystems, open oceans or extreme environments (extremophiles). This field includes other branches of microbiology such as: microbial ecology (microbially-mediated nutrient cycling), geomicrobiology, (microbial diversity), water microbiology (the study of those microorganisms that are found in water), aeromicrobiology (the study of airborne microorganisms) and epidemiology (the study of the incidence, spread, and control of disease).

This is by no means an exhaustive list of the different types of applied microbiology, but gives an indication of the expansive variety of the field and some of the benefits these studies entail.

KEY POINTS

Using knowledge gained by microbiologists studying microbes, several fields of applied microbiology have formed.

While food and medicinal applications is a big portion of applied microbiology, the study of microbes has led to entire commercial industries which affect almost all aspects of human life.

There are a myriad of practical applications that microbiology contributes to, including several parts of food production and medicinal applications.

TERMS

rhizosphere
The soil region subject to the influence of plant roots and their associated microorganisms.

biotechnology
The use of living organisms (especially microorganisms) in industrial, agricultural, medical, and other technological applications.

pathogenic
Able to cause harmful disease.

ANTISEPTICS AND ANTIBIOTICS

Surprisingly, most microbes are not harmful to humans. In fact, they are all around us and even a part of us. However, some microbes are human pathogens; to combat these, we use immunization, antiseptics, and antibiotics.
Immunization is the process by which an individual's immune system becomes fortified against an agent (known as the immunogen).

When the immune system is exposed to molecules that are foreign to the body, it will orchestrate an immune response. It will also develop the ability to respond quickly to subsequent encounters with the same substance, a phenomenon known as immunological memory. Therefore, by exposing a person to an immunogen in a controlled way, the body can learn to protect itself: this is called active immunization.

Vaccines against microorganisms that cause diseases can prepare the body's immune system, thus helping it fight or prevent an infection. The most important elements of the immune system that are improved by immunization are the T cells, the B cells, and the antibodies B cells produce. Memory B cells and memory T cells are responsible for the swift response to a second encounter with a foreign molecule. Through the use of immunizations, some infections and diseases have been almost completely eradicated throughout the United States and the world. For example, polio was eliminated in the U.S. in 1979. Active immunization and vaccination has been named one of the "Ten Great Public Health Achievements in the 20th Century".

By contrast, in *passive* immunization, pre-synthesized elements of the immune system are transferred to a human body so it does not need to produce these elements itself. Currently, antibodies can be used for passive immunization. This method of immunization starts to work very quickly; however, it is short-lasting because the antibodies are naturally broken down and will disappear altogether if there are no B cells to produce more of them. Passive immunization occurs physiologically, when antibodies are transferred from mother to fetus during pregnancy, to protect the fetus before and shortly after birth. The antibodies can be produced in animals, called "serum therapy," although there is a high chance of anaphylactic shock because of immunity against animal serum itself. Thus, humanized antibodies produced *in vitro* by cell culture are used instead if available.

In early inquiries before there was an understanding of microbes, much emphasis was given to the prevention of putrefaction. Procedures were carried out to determine the amount of agent that needed to be added to a given solution in order to prevent the development of pus and putrefaction. However, due to a lack of understanding of germ theory, this method was inaccurate. Today, an antiseptic is judged by its effect on pure cultures of a defined microbe or on their vegetative and spore forms.

Antiseptics are antimicrobial substances that are applied to living tissue to reduce the possibility of infection, sepsis, or putrefaction. Their earliest known systematic use was in the ancient practice of embalming the dead. Antiseptics are generally distinguished from antibiotics by the latter's ability to be transported through the lymphatic system to destroy bacteria within the body, and from disinfectants, which destroy microorganisms found on non-living objects. Some antiseptics are true germicides, capable of destroying microbes (bacteriocidal), while others are bacteriostatic and only prevent or inhibit bacterial growth. Microbicides that destroy virus particles are called viricides or antivirals.

An antibacterial is a compound or substance that kills or slows down the growth of bacteria. The term is often used synonymously with the term antibiotic; today, however, with increased knowledge of the causative agents of various infectious diseases, the term "antibiotic" has come to denote a broader range of antimicrobial compounds, including anti-fungal and other compounds.

The word "antibiotic" was first used in 1942 by Selman Waksman and his collaborators to describe any substance produced by a microorganism that is antagonistic to the growth of other microorganisms in high dilution. This definition excluded substances that kill bacteria but are not produced by microorganisms (such as gastric juices and hydrogen peroxide). It also excluded synthetic antibacterial compounds, such as the sulfonamides. Many antibacterial compounds are relatively small molecules with a molecular weight of less than 2000 amu. With advances in medicinal chemistry, most of today's antibacterials are semisynthetic modifications of various natural compounds.

KEY POINTS

Immunization is the fortification of our own immune system, priming it against potential future infections by specific microbes.
Antiseptics are broadly defined as substances we can use on our body or surfaces around us to slow or kill microbes that could potentially harm us.
Antibiotics, like antiseptics, can slow or kill microbes. However, unlike antiseptics, antibiotics can circulate in the human blood system and be used to fight microbial infections.

TERMS

immunogen
any substance that elicits a immune response; an antigen

anaphylactic shock
A severe and rapid systemic allergic reaction to an allergen, constricting the trachea and preventing breathing.

MICROBIOLOGY TERMS

Abiotic Factors
Non-living factors that can affect life, like soil, nutrients, climate, wind etc.

Absorption Field
An organized system of meticulously constructed narrow trenches, which are partially filled with washed gravel or crushed stone, into which a pipe is placed. Discharges from septic tanks are passed through these trenches.

Acetogenic Bacterium
An aerobic, gram negative bacteria, that is rod-shaped, which is made of non-sporogenous organisms that produce acetic acid as a waste product.

Acetylene Block Assay
Determines the release of nitrous oxide gas from acetylene treated soil, which is used to estimate denitrification.

Acetylene Reduction Assay
This is used to estimate nitrogenase activity by measuring the rate of reduction of ethylene to acetylene.

Acid Soil
Soil which has a pH value lesser than 6.6

Acidophile
An organism that grows well in an acidic medium (up to a pH of 1).

Actinomycete
These are Gram positive, nonmotile, nonsporing, noncapsulated filaments that break into bacillary and coccoid elements. They resemble fungi, and most are free living, particularly in soil.

Actinorhizae
The association present between actinomycetes and roots of plants.

Activated Sludge
Sludge particles which are produced in raw or settled wastewater, by the growth of organisms in aeration tanks. This is all done in the presence of dissolved oxygen. This sludge contains living organisms that can feed on incoming wastewater

Activation Energy
The amount of energy required to bring all molecules in one mole of a substance, to their reactive state, at a given temperature

Active Carrier
An infected person who has visible clinical symptoms of a disease, and is capable of transmitting the disease to other individuals.

Active Site
The location on the surface of the enzyme where the substrate binds.

Adjuvant
The material added to an antigen to increase its immunogenicity, for example, alum

Aerobic
This includes organisms that require molecular oxygen to survive (aerobic organisms), an environment that has molecular oxygen, and processes that happen only in the presence of oxygen (aerobic respiration).

Aerobic Anoxygenic Photosynthesis
Photosynthetic process which takes place under aerobic conditions, but which does not result in the formation of oxygen.

Aerotolerant Anaerobes
Microbes that can survive in both, aerobic and anaerobic conditions, because they obtain their energy by fermentation.

Aflatoxin
A toxin produced by Aspergillus flavus and Aspergillus parasiticus, which contaminate groundnut seedlings. This is said to be a cause of hepatic carcinoma.

Agar
A dried hydrophilic, colloidal substance extracted from red algae species, used as a solid culture media for bacteria and other micro-organisms. Also used as a bulk laxative, in making emulsions and as a supporting medium for immunodiffusion and immunoelectrophoresis

Agarose
Agarose is obtained from seaweed and is used as a resolving medium in electrophoresis. It consists of non-sulfated linear polymer, which contains D-galactose and 3:6-anhydro-L-galactose alternately.

Agglutinates
The visible clumps that are formed as a result of an agglutination reaction.

Agglutination Reaction
The process of clumping together, in suspension of antigen bearing cells, micro-organisms, or particles in the presence of specific antibodies called agglutinins. This leads to the formation of an insoluble immune complex.

Airborne Transmission
A type of transmission, wherein the organism is suspended in or spreads its infection by air.

Akinete
A resting non-motile, dormant, thick-walled spore state of cyanobacteria and algae

Alcoholic Fermentation
A fermentation process that produces alcohol (ethanol) and carbon dioxide from sugars.

Alga
Phototrophic eukaryotic micro-organisms, that maybe unicellular or multicellular. These include phaeophyta: brown algae, spirogyra and red algae.

Aliphatic
Pertaining to any member of one of the two major groups of organic compounds, with the main carbon structure as a straight chain

Alkaline Soil
Soil having pH greater than 7.3.

Alkalophile
Organisms that have an affinity for alkaline media, thus, growing best in such conditions

Allochthonous Flora
Organisms that are not originally found in soil, but reach there by precipitation, sewage, diseased tissue and other such means. They do not contribute much ecologically.

Allosteric Site
A non-active site on the enzyme body, where a non-substrate compound binds. This may result in conformational changes at the active site.

Allotype
Any of various allelic variants of a protein, characterized by antigenic differences.

Alpha Hemolysis
A partial clearing zone, greenish in color, around a bacterial colony that grows on blood agar.

Alpha-proteobacteria
One of the five sub-groups of proteobacteria, each with distinctive 16S rRNA sequences. Mostly contains oligotrophic proteobacteria, many of which have distinctive morphological features.

Alternative Complement Pathway
A pathway of complement activation, including the C3-C9 components of the classical pathway. It is independent of antibody activity.

Alveolar Macrophage

A highly active and aggressive phagocytic macrophage, located on the epithelial lining of the lung alveoli, which ingests and destroys any inhaled particles and micro-organisms.

Amensalism (Antagonism)
A type of symbiosis, wherein one population is adversely affected, while the other is unaffected

Ames Test
A test that uses a special strain of salmonella to test chemicals for mutagenicity and carcinogenicity

Amino Acid Activation
The first stage of synthesis of proteins, where the amino acid is attached to transfer RNA.

Amino Group
The monovalent radical NH2, attached to a carbon skeleton, as seen in amines and amino acids.

Aminoacyl or Acceptor Site (A site)
The site on the ribosome that contains an aminoacyl-tRNA at the beginning of the elongation cycle during protein synthesis.

Ammonia Oxidation
A test which is conducted during manufacturing process, to evaluate ammonia oxidation rate for nitrifiers.

Ammonification
Liberation of ammonia by micro-organisms acting on organic nitrogenous compounds

Amoeba
A minute protozoan, occurring as a single cell with a nucleus, that changes shape by extruding its cytoplasm, leading to the formation of pseudopodia, by means of which it absorbs food and moves

Amoeboid Movement
Movement by means of extrusions of the cytoplasm, leading to formation of foot-like processes called pseudopodia.

Amphibolic Pathways
Metabolic pathways that function both anabolically, as well as catabolically.

Amphitrichous
A cell which has a single flagellum at each end

Amphotericin B
An antibiotic derived from streptomyces nodosus which is effective against many species of fungi and certain species of leishmania.

Anaerobic

Refers to organisms that survive in the absence of oxygen (anearobic organisms), the absence of molecular oxygen, processes occurring in the absence of oxygen like anearobic respiration.

Anamorph
A stage of fungal reproduction, where cells are asexually formed by the process of mitosis.

Anaplerotic Reactions
Reactions that help replenish intermediates in the tricarboxylic acid cycle when their reserves are depleted.

Anergy
Decreased responsiveness to antigens, to the extent that there is an inability to react to substances that are expected to be antigenic

Anion Exchange Capacity
Total exchangeable anions that a soil can adsorb. The unit used to express the amount is in centimoles of negative charge per kilogram of soil.

Annotation
The process of determining the exact location of specific genes in a genome map

Anoxic
A condition or state which is devoid of oxygen.

Anoxygenic Photosynthesis
A type of photosynthesis where oxygen is not produced. This phenomenon is seen in green and purple bacteria.

Antagonist
A drug that binds to a hormone, neurotransmitter, or another drug, thus, blocking the action of the other substance.

Antheridium
The male gametangium found in phylum Oomycota (kingdom Stramenopila) and phylum Ascomyta (kingdom Fungi)

Anthrax
An often fatal and infectious disease, caused by ingestion or inhalation of spores of Bacillus anthracis, which are normally found in soil. It is acquired by humans through contaminated wool or animal products or by inhalation of airborne spores

Anthropogenic
Something that is derived from human activities.

Antibiosis

Lysis of an organism brought about by metabolic products of the antagonist. This can be caused by enzymes, lytic agents or other toxic compounds

Antibiotic
A chemical substance produced by a microorganism, which has the capacity to inhibit the growth of, or kill other micro-organisms

Antibody
An immunoglobulin molecule that reacts with a specific antigen that induced its synthesis and with molecules that have a similar structure

Antibody-Dependent Cell-Mediated Cytotoxicity (ADCC)
A type of reaction wherein, cells with Fc receptors that recognize the Fc region of the bound antibody, kill the antibody-coated target cells.

Anticodon Triplet
A triplet of nucleotides in transfer RNA that is complementary to the codon in messenger RNA.

Antigen
Any substance capable of instigating the immune system into action, inciting a specific immune response and of reacting with the products of that response.

Antimetabolite
A substance that interferes with a specific metabolic pathway, by inhibiting a key enzyme, due its resemblance with the normal enzyme substrate.

Antimicrobial Agent
An agent that has the capacity to kill or inhibit the growth of micro-organisms

Antisense RNA
One of the strands of a double-stranded molecule, which does not directly encode the product, but is complementary to it, thus, inhibiting its activity.

Antiseptic
A substance that inhibits the growth and development of micro-organisms, but does not necessarily kill them.

Aplanospore
A spore that is formed during asexual reproduction, which is nonflagellated and nonmotile.

Apoenzyme
A protein part of an enzyme that is separable from the prosthetic group (the coenzyme).

Apoptosis
A pattern of cell death which is often called 'programmed death' or 'suicide of cells', wherein the cell breaks up into fragments, which are membrane bound. These fragments are then eliminated

by phagocytosis. This is a protective mechanism, by which the cell prevents spread of infection to other cells by sacrificing itself.

Aporepressor
A product of regulator genes, that combines with the corepressor to form the complete repressor.

Arbuscule
Special structure formed in the root cortical cells by arbuscular mycorrhizal fungi. The structure formed resembles a tree.

Artificially Acquired Passive Immunity
A type of temporary immunity that results from the introduction of antibodies produced by another organism or by in vitro methods, into the body.

Aseptic Technique
Procedures that are performed under strict sterile conditions. These procedures maybe laboratory procedures such as microbiological cultures.

Assimilatory Nitrate Reduction
Reduction of nitrate to compounds like ammonium, for the synthesis of amino acids and proteins.

Associative Dinitrogen Fixation
An enhanced rate of dinitrogen fixation, brought about by a close relationship between free-living diazotrophic organisms and a higher plant.

Associative Symbiosis
Interaction between two dissimilar organisms or biological systems, which is normally mutually beneficial.

Autogenous Infection
An infection which occurs due to the microbiota of the patient himself.

Autoimmune Disease
A disease where the target is the body's own tissues, that is, there is attacking of self-antigens.

Autoimmunity
A condition where a specific humoral or cell mediated immune response is initiated against the constituents of the body's own tissues. It normally leads to hypersesitivity reactions, and if it persists, can even escalate to an autoimmune disease.

Autolysins
A lysin that originates in an organism, which is capable of destroying its own cells and tissues.

Autoradiography

Making a radiograph of an object or tissue by recording the radiation emitted by it on a photographic plate. The radiation is emitted by radioactive material within the object or tissue.

Autotrophic Nitrification
The combined nitrification action of two autotrophic organisms, one converting ammonium to nitrite and the other oxidizing nitrite to nitrate.

Auxotroph
A mutated type of organism that requires specific organic growth factors, in addition to the carbon source present in a minimal medium.

Axenic
Pure cultures of micro-organisms, that is, which are not contaminated by any foreign organisms.

Axial Filament
Found in spirochetes, it is the organ of motility.

B-cell (B lymphocyte)
Bursa-dependent lymphocytes which are precursors of antibody-producing cells (plasma cells) and the cells primarily responsible for humoral immunity.

B-cell Antigen Receptor (BCR)
The membrane which is formed of membrane immunoglobulin or surface immunoglobulin, which allows a B-cell to detect, when a specific antigen is present in the body, and triggers B-cell activation.

Bacteria
A domain that contains prokaryotic cells that are not multicellular. Read more on bacteria.

Bacteremia
Presence of bacteria in the blood.

Bacterial Artificial Chromosome
A cloning vector that is derived from E. coli, which is used to clone foreign DNA fragments in E. coli.

Bacterial Photosynthesis
A mode of metabolism, which is light-dependent and where carbon dioxide is reduced to glucose, which is used for energy production and biosynthesis. It is an anaerobic reaction.

Bactericide
A substance that kills bacteria

Bacteriochlorophyll
A light absorbing pigment found in phototrophic bacteria, like green sulfur and purple sulfur bacteria.

Bacteriocin
Substances that are produced by bacteria which kill other strains of bacteria by inducing a metabolic block.

Bacteriorhodopsin
A protein involved in light mediated ATP synthesis, which contains retinal. It is one of the main characteristics of archaebacteria.

Bacteriostatic
An agent that inhibits the growth or multiplication of bacteria, but does not kill them.

Bacteroid
A genus of bacteroides, these are Gram negative, rod-shaped, anaerobic bacteria which are normal inhabitants of the oral, respiratory, urogenital and intestinal cavities of animals and humans.

Baeocytes
Reproductive cells formed by cyanobacteria through multiple fission. They are small and spherical in shape.

Balanced Growth
Microbial growth where all cellular constituents are synthesized at constant rates, in relation to each other.

Barophile
An organism that thrives in conditions of high hydrostatic pressure.

Barotolerant
An organism that can tolerate high hydrostatic pressure, although it will grow better under normal pressure.

Basal Body
A cylindrical structure that attaches the flagella to the cell body at the base of prokaryotic or eukaryotic organisms.

Basal Medium
A basal medium allows the growth of many types of micro-organisms which do not require special nutrient supplements.

Base Composition
The proportion of total bases consisting of guanine plus cytosine or thymine plus adenine base pairs.

Basidioma
Fruiting body that produces the basidia.

Basidiospore
The sexual spore of the Basidiomycotina, which is formed on the basidium.

Batch Culture
A culture of micro-organisms which is obtained by inoculating a dish containing a single batch of medium.

Batch Process
A treatment procedure wherein, a tank or reactor is filled, the solution is treated, and the tank is emptied. Batch processes are mostly used to cleanse, stabilize, or condition chemical solutions for use in industries.

Benthic Zone
The ecological region at the lowest level of a water body, including the sediment surface and some sub-surface layers.

Beta Hemolysis
A clear zone seen around a bacterial colony growing on blood agar.

Bio-Tower
A tower filled with a media similar to a rachet or plastic rings, where air and water are forced up the tower by a counterflow movement. It is an attached culture system.

Bioaccumulation
Intracellular accumulation of chemical substances in living tissue.

Bioaugmentation
Addition to the micro-organism's environment that can metabolize and grow on specific organic compounds.

Bioavailability
The extent to which a drug or other substance becomes available to the target tissue after administration.

Biochemical Oxygen Demand
The amount of dissolved oxygen consumed in five days by biological processes breaking down organic matter. It is a test that measures the oxygen consumed (in mg/L) over five days at 20 degrees Celsius.

Biodegradable
The property by which a substance is capable of being degraded by biological processes, like bacterial or enzymatic action.

Biodegradation

The process of breakdown of substances by chemical reactions, thus rendering these substances less harmful to the environment.

Bioinsecticide
A pathogen (either bacteria, virus or fungi) used to kill or inhibit the activity of unwanted insect pests.

Bioluminescence
The production of light in living organisms by the enzyme luciferase.

Biomagnification
Increase in the concentration of a chemical substance, as its position progresses in the food chain.

Biostimulation
A process which helps catalyze the activity of micro-organisms involved in biodegradation

Biosynthesis
Production of cellular constituents from simpler compounds.

Biotransformation
The chemical alterations of a drug, occurring in the body, due to enzymatic activity.

Biotrophic
Close associations seen between two different organisms, that work mutually to benefit each other.

Bioventing
A procedure where the subsurface is aerated to enhance biological activity of naturally occurring micro-organisms in the soil.

Blastomycosis
An infection caused due to Blastomyces dermatitidis, it predominantly affects skin, lungs and bones.

Burst size
The number of phages ejected by a host cell over the course of its lytic life cycle.

Butanediol Fermentation
A kind of fermentation found in Enterobacteriaceae family, where 2,3-Butanediol is a major product.

Capsid
The outer proteinaceous coat of a virus.

Capsomere

A protein sub-unit of the capsid of a virus.

Carbon Cycle
The cycle where carbon-dioxide is taken in and converted to organic compunds by photosynthesis or chemosynthesis, after which it is partially incorporated into sediments, and then returned to the atmosphere by respiration or combustion

Carbon Fixation
Conversion of carbon-dioxide and other single carbon compounds to organic compunds such as carbohydrates.

Carbon-Nitrogen (C/N) ratio
Ratio of carbon mass to nitrogen mass in soil or other organic material.

Carboxyl Group
The -COOH group found attached to the main carbon skeleton in certain compounds, like carboxylic acids and fatty acids.

Carboxysomes
Polyhedral cell inclusions which form the key enzyme of the Calvin cycle.

Carcinogen
An often mutated substance which is implicated as one of the causing agents of cancer.

Catabolism
A process by which complex substances are broken down into simpler compounds, often accompanied by the release of energy.

Catabolite Repression
Transcription-level inhibition of inducible enzymes by glucose, or other easily available carbon sources.

Cell-mediated Immunity
Immunity resulting from destruction of foreign organisms and infected cells by the active action of T-lymphocytes on them. It can be acquired by individuals by the transfer of cells.

Cellular Slime Molds
Slime molds with a vegetative phase containing amoeboid cells that come together to form a pseudoplasmodium.

Cellulitis
A diffused inflammation of the soft or connective tissue, in which a thin and watery exudate spreads through tissue spaces, often leading to ulceration and abscess formation.

Cephalosporin

A group of broad-spectrum, penicillinase resistant antibiotics, derived from Cephalosporium. Read more on different types of antibiotics.

Chaperonin
Heat shock proteins that oversee correct folding and assembly of polypeptides in bacteria, plasmids, eukaryotic, cytosol, and mitochondria.

Chelate
A chemical compound in which a metallic ion is firmly bound into a ring within the chelating molecule. Chelates are used in metal poisoning.

Chemoautotroph
Organisms that obtain their enegry from the oxidation of inorganic chemicals and other carbon compounds.

Chemoheterotroph
Organisms that obtain energy and carbon from the oxidation of organic compunds.

Chemolithotroph
Living organisms that obtain their energy from oxidation of inorganic compunds, which act as electron donors.

Chemoorganotroph
Organisms that obtain energy and electrons from the oxidation of organic compounds.

Chemostat
A continuously used culture device, controlled by limited amounts of nutrients and dilution rates.

Chemotaxis
Movement of a motile organism under the influence of a chemical. It maybe attracted towards the chemical or maybe repulsed by it.

Chemotrophs
Organisms that obtain their energy by the oxidation of chemical compounds.

Chlamydospore
A thick walled intercalary or terminal asexual spore which is not shed. It is formed by rounding up of a cell.

Chronic Carrier
An individual carrying a pathogen over an extended period of time.

Chytrid
A fungus belonging to the genus Chytridomycota. It is spherical in shape and has rhizoids, which are short, thin filamentous branches, that resemble fine roots.

Cilia
Minute hairlike extensions present on a cell surface, which move in a rhythmic manner.

Ciliate
A protozoan that moves with the help of cilia.

Clarification
The process of purification of water, where suspended material in the water is removed. It can be done by using sedimentation, filtration or by the use of adsorbing chemicals like alum.

Clone
Cells which have descended from a single parent cell. Organisms having identical copies of DNA structure, which is obtained by replication.

Colonization
Establishment of an entire community of micro-organisms at a designated site.

Colorless Sulfur Bacteria
A group of nonphotosynthetic bacteria that oxidize sulfur compounds, thus deriving their energy by this process.

Combinatorial Biology
The process of transfer of genetic material from one microorganism to another. Mostly used to synthesize products such as antibiotics. It is also used in genetic engineering.

Cometabolism
Transformation of a substrate by a microorganism without deriving energy or nutrients from the substrate.

Competent
The ability to take up DNA.

Complementary DNA
A DNA copy of any RNA molecule, like mRNA or tRNA

Complex Viruses
Viruses with capsids that are neither icosahedral nor helical. They have a complicated symmetry.

Conditional Mutations
Mutations occurring only under certain specific conditions.

Conidiospore
A thin-walled, asexual spore seen on hyphae which is not contained in sporangium.

Conjugants

Mating partners that participate in conjugation, which is a type of sexual reproduction, seen in protozoans.

Conjugative Plasmid
A self transmissible plasmid, or a plasmid that can encode all functions required to bring about its conjugation.

Consortium
Two or more members working together, where each organism benefits from the other, thus often performing functions that may not be possible to carry out individually.

Constitutive Enzyme
Enzymes synthesized in the cell, irrespective of the environmental conditions surrounding the cell.

Cosmid
A plasmid vector which can be packed in a phage capsid. It is useful for cloning large fragments of DNA.

Cyanobacterium
A photosynthetic, nitrogen fixing bacteria which includes the blue-green bacteria.

Cyst
Resting stage of certain bacteria and protozoans, wherein the entire cell is surrounded by a protective layer.

Cytokine
Non-antibody proteins released by a cell when it comes in contact with specific antigens.

Cytoplasm
The protoplasm of a cell, exclusive of the nucleus. Read more on the structure and functions of cytoplasm.

Cytoplasmic Membrane
A selectively permeable membrane which is present around the cytoplasm of the cell.

Decomposition
Chemical breakdown of a compound into smaller and simpler compounds by micro-organisms.

Defined Medium
A medium whose quantitative and chemical composition is exactly known.

Degradation
Process by which a compound is transformed into simpler compounds.

Denaturation

Process by which double stranded DNA unwinds into two single strands.

Denitrification
Reduction of nitrate or nitrite into simpler nitrogenous compounds like molecular nitrogen or nitrogen oxides.

Derepressible Enzyme
Enzyme produced in the absence of a specific inhibitory compound.

Dew point
The temperature to which air must be cooled to bring about the condensation of water vapor.

Diazotroph
Organism capable of using dinitrogen as its sole nitrogen source.

Differential Medium
A medium with certain indicators, which helps distinguish between different chemical reactions during growth of organisms on it.

Diffused Air Aeration
A diffused air activated sludge plant takes air, compresses it and discharges it with force, below the surface of water.

Dikaryon
When two nuclei are present in the same hyphal compartment (they maybe homokaryon or heterokaryon), it is known as dikaryon.

Dilution Plate Count Method
A method of estimating the number of viable micro-organisms in a sample.

Dinitrogen Fixation
Conversion of molecular dinitrogen into ammonia and other organic combinations useful in other biological processes.

Direct Count
Using direct microscopic examination to determine the number of micro-organisms present in a given mass of soil.

Disinfectant
An agent that kills micro-organisms.

DNA Fingerprinting
Techniques by which possible differences between different DNA samples can be assessed.

Dolipore Septum
Specialized cross-wall that separates hypha of fungi belonging to the genus Basidiomycota.

Domain
The highest level of biological classification which goes beyond kingdoms. The three domains of biological organisms are Bacteria, Eukarya, and Archaea.

Doubling Time
The time needed for a certain population to double in number.

Endoenzyme
Enzyme that acts along the internal portion of a polymer.

Endonuclease
The endoenzyme responsible for breaking the phosphodiester bonds in a nucleic acid molecule.

Endophyte
An organism, which maybe parasitic or symbiotic, with a plant that is grown within.

Endospore
A cell which is formed by certain gram-positive bacteria in unfavorable conditions. An endospore is extremely resistant to heat and other harmful agents.

Enhanced Rhizosphere Degradation
Enhanced activity of micro-organisms involved with biodegradation of contaminants near plant roots which is brought about by compounds exuded by the plant roots.

Enrichment Culture
Technique wherein environmental conditions are altered to aid the growth of a specific organism or group of organisms.

Enteric Bacteria
These are bacteria present in the intestinal tract of humans and other animals. They maybe physiologic or pathologic.

Episome
An extrachromosomal replicating genetic element found in certain bacteria.

Epitope
An antigenic determinant of known structure. It is the region of the antigen to which the variable region of the antibody binds.

Ericoid Mycorrhizae
The type of mycorrhizae found in Ericales plants. These hyphae are capable of penetrating cortical cells.

Estuaries
Water bodies located at river ends. They are subjected to tidal fluctuations.

Eubacteria
A genus of bacteria belonging to the family Propionibacteriaceae, found as saprophytes in soil and water.

Exoenzyme
An enzyme which acts outside the cell that secretes it.

Exons
The region of a split DNA that codes for RNA.

Extracellular
Outside the cell.

Exudate
A fluid high in protein and cellular debris which has escaped from blood vessels, usually as a result of inflammation.

Facultative Organism
An organism which is able to adjust to a particular circumstance or has the ability to take up different roles in a process.

Feedback Initiation
Inhibition by an end product of the biosynthetic pathway involved in its synthesis.

Fertilizer
Any organic or inorganic material added to the soil to enhance the growth of plants.

Field Capacity
Content of water remaining in the soil after being saturated with water.

Filamentous
In the form of very long rods, mostly seen in bacteria. Seen as branching strands in fungi.

Fimbria
Short filamentous structure present on a bacterial cell, involved with adhesion of the bacteria to other surfaces it comes in contact with.

Frustule
Siliceous wall and protoplasm seen in diatoms.

Fulvic Acid
The yellow organic material that remains behind after removal of humic acid by the process of acidification.

Fungistasis

Suppression of growth of new fungal cells, due to excessive competition for nutrients, or due to the presence of excessive inhibitory compounds in the soil.

Fungus
Eukaryotic heterotrophic organisms that live as saprophytes or parasites. This group includes mushrooms, yeast and molds. They have a rigid cell wall.

Fluorescent Antibody
This is a laboratory test that is done, wherein antibodies are tagged with fluorescent dye to detect the presence of micro-organisms.

Gas Vacuole
A sub-cellular organelle, found only in prokaryotes, which are gas filled vesicles.

Gene Cloning
Isolation of a desired gene from an organism and its replication in large amounts. It is used extensively in DNA research.

Gene Probe
A strand of nucleic acid which can be labeled and hybridized to a complementary molecule from a mixture of other nucleic acids. It is helpful in DNA sequencing.

Generation Time
The time required for a population to double in number.

Genetic Code
The information on the DNA, which is required for the synthesis of proteins.

Glycosidase
The enzyme responsible for hydrolizing a glucosidic linkage between two sugar molecules.

Gram Stain
A differential stain that divides bacteria into two groups, as Gram positive and Gram negative, depending on the ability of the organism to retain crystal violet when decolorized with an organic solvent like ethanol.

Growth
An increase in the number of cells, and the size and constituents present in the cells.

Growth Factor
Organic compound essential for growth which is required in trace amounts, and which cannot be synthesized by the organism itself.

Growth Rate
The rate at which growth occurs.

Growth Rate Constant
Slope of log10 of the number of cells per unit volume plotted against time.

Growth Yield Coefficient
Quantity of carbon formed per unit of substrate carbon consumed.

Halophile
An organism that thrives, or at least which can survive in a saline environment.

Halotolerant
An organism that can survive in a saline environment, but does not require a saline environment for growth.

Hapten
A substance not inducing antibody formation, but which is able to combine with a specific antibody.

Heterokaryon
Hypha that contains at least two genetically dissimilar nuclei.

Heterolactic Fermentation
A kind of lactic acid fermentation, wherein various sugars are fermented into different products.

Heterothallic
Hyphae that are incompatible with each other, thus requiring another compatible hypha to mate with, to form a dikaryon or a diploid.

Heterotrophic Nitrification
The oxidation of ammonium to nitrite and nitrate by heterotrophic organisms.

Hexose Monophosphate Pathway
A metabolic pathway involving the oxidative decarboxylation of glucose:6:phosphate.

Holomictic
These are those lakes, wherein the water in them at some point of time will have a uniform temperature and density from top to bottom, thus allowing the lake waters to mix completely.

Holomorph
A fungus which consists of all sexual and asexual stages in its life cycle.

Homofermentation
A type of fermentation where there is only one type of end product generated.

Homokaryon
A fungal hypha containing nuclei which are genetically identical.

Homolactic Fermentation
A type of lactic acid fermentation, in which all sugars involved are converted into lactic acid.

Homothallic
Hyphae that are self-compatible, that is, sexual reproduction occurs in the same organism by meiosis and genetic recombination. Fusion of these hyphae lead to the formation of dikaryon or diploid.

Host
An organism that can harbor or nourish another organism.

Heterofermentation
Any fermentation where there is more than one main end product.

Humic Acid
Dark colored organic material extracted from the soil by the use of reagents and which is precipitated by acid.

Humic Substances
High molecular weight substances formed by secondary synthesis reactions, for example, humic acid and fulvic acid.

Humification
The process of conversion of organic residues into humic substances by biochemical processes.

Hybridization
Natural or artificial construction of a duplex nucleic acid molecule by complementary base pairing between two nucleic acid strands derived from different sources.

Hydrocarbon
An organic compound containing carbon and hydrogen only.

Hydrogen Oxidizing Bacterium
These are bacteria that oxidize hydrogen for energy and synthesize carbohydrates, using carbon dioxide as their source of carbon in the absence of other organic compounds.

Hyperparasite
Parasite that feeds on another parasite.

Hyperthermophile
An organism that thrives in temperatures ranging around 80 degrees Celsius or more.

Hypolimnion
This is the dense, bottom layer of water, that lies below the thermocline, in a thermally stratified lake.

Illuviation
Repositioning of soil removed from one horizon to another.

Immobilization
Conversion of an element from inorganic to organic form.

Immunity
The protection mechanism against infections caused by micro-organisms or toxins, that is inherent in the body.

Immunoblot
The technique for analyzing or identifying proteins via antigen:antibody specific reactions.

Immunofluoresence
The technique to determine the location of an antigen or antibody in a tissue section or smear by fluorescence.

Immunogen
A substance that has the capacity to bring about an immune response.

Immunoglobulin
A protein which has antibody activity.

In vivo
Inside the body.

Inducible Enzyme
An enzyme generated in response to an external factor.

Infection
Invasion and multiplication of micro-organisms in body tissues, leading to various diseases and disorders.

Infection Thread
The tube in root hair, through which rhizobia reach and infect roots.

Infrared (IR)
The portion of the electromagnetic spectrum whose wavelength ranges from 0.75 microns to 1 millimeter.

Inoculate
To treat a medium with micro-organisms for the purpose of creating a favorable response.

Inoculum
The material used to introduce an organism into a certain medium for growth.

Insertion
A type of genetic mutation, wherein single or multiple nucleotides are added to DNA.

Insertion Sequence
The simplest possible type of transposable elements.

Integration
The process by which a DNA molecule becomes incorporated into another genome.

Interspecies Hydrogen Transfer
The process of hydrogen production and consumption reactions, occurring by the interaction of various micro-organisms.

Intracellular
Inside the cell.

Isoenzyme
When two different enzymes, which may be different in their composition, act as catalysts for the same reaction, or set of reactions.

Isolation
A procedure wherein a pure culture of an organism is obtained from a sample or an environment.

Isomorphous Substitution
The substitution of an atom by a similarly sized atom of lower valence, in a crystalline clay sheet.

Jaccard's Coefficient
An association coefficient of numerical taxonomy, which is the proportion of characters that match, excluding those that both organisms lack.

K- Strategy
Ecological strategy where organisms depend on adapting physiologically to the resources available in their immediate environment.

Koch's Postulates
Laws given by Robert Koch which prove that an organism is the causative agent of a disease.

Lag Phase
The time period when there is no increase in the number of micro-organisms, seen after inoculation of fresh growth medium.

Lamella
Seen in plants as the layers of protoplasmic membranes in chloroplast that contain photosynthetic pigments.

Leaching
Removal of metals from ores by the help of micro-organisms.

Lectins
Plant proteins with a high affinity for specific sugar residues.

Leghemoglobin
Red colored pigments rich in iron, which are produced in root nodules during symbiotic association between rhizobia and leguminous plants.

Ligand
A molecule, ion or group of molecules or ions, bound to the central atom by means of a chelate or coordination compound.

Light Compensation Point
The point where the rate of respiration is higher than the rate of photosynthesis, which usually occurs at about 1% of sunlight intensity.

Lime (agricultural)
Soil **amendment containing** high levels of calcium compounds, like calcium carbonate and other such mineral which are used to neutralize soil acidity, and provide calcium for plant growth.

Lipopolysaccharide (LPS)
Complex lipid structure containing sugars and fatty acids, which is commonly found in most Gram negative bacteria.

Lithotroph
An organism that uses inorganic substrate such as ammonia or hydrogen to act as electron donors in energy metabolism. They maybe chemolithotrophs or photolithotrophs.

Litter
The surface layer of forests which is laden with leaves, twigs, fruits etc.

Lophotrichous
An organism that has a tuft of flagella that is polar in nature.

Luxury Uptake
Uptake of nutrients in excess of what is required by an organism for its normal growth.

Lysis
The rupture and destruction of a cell, resulting in loss of cellular contents.

Lysogeny
An association where a prokaryote contains a prophage and the virus genome is replicated in sync with the chromosome of the host.

Lysosome
A cell organelle which contains lytic enzymes.

Macronutrient
A substance required in large amounts for normal growth of an individual.

Macropore
Larger soil pores from which water drains readily by gravity.

Magnetosome
Small particles of magnetite, which is a compound containing magnesium, present in cells that exhibit magnetotaxis.

Magnetotactic Bacteria
Bacteria that orient themselves according to the earth's magnetic field due to the presence of the magnetosomes.

Manure
Animal excreta, with or without a bedding of litter at various stages of decomposition. It's normally considered to be a good fertilizer.

Mass Flow (nutrient)
The movement of solutes in relation to the movement of water.

Medium
A source where micro-organisms are grown.

Mesofauna
Animals residing in the soil which are 200 to 1000 microns in length. This group includes nematodes, oligochaete worms, smaller insect larvae and certain anthropods.

Mesophile
An organism that thrives in temperatures ranging from 15 - 40 degrees Celsius.

Methanogenesis
The production of methane by biological reactions.

Methanogenic Bacterium
Bacteria that produce methane as a by-product of their chemical reactions.

Methanotroph
An organism capable of oxidizing methane.

Microaerophile

Micro-organisms that grow well in relatively low oxygen concentration environments.

Microaggregate
Clusters of clay stabilized by organic matter and precipitated inorganic matter.

Microbial Biomass
Total mass of micro-organisms living in a given mass or volume of soil.

Microbial Population
Total number of micro-organisms living in a given mass or volume of soil.

Microbiology
The study of micro-organisms, often with the aid of a microscope.

Microcosm
A community or any other unit that is representative of a larger community.

Microenvironment
The immediate physical and chemical surroundings of a microorganism.

Microfauna
Protozoa, nematodes and anthropods that are smaller than 200 microns.

Microflora
This includes bacteria, virus, fungi and algae.

Micrometer
One millionth of a meter (10^{-6} meters).

Micronutrient
Elements that are required for growth in trace amounts. These include copper, iron, zinc etc.

Micro-organism
An organism that is too small to be seen by the naked eye. Also called microbes, these include bacteria, fungi, protozoans, algae and viruses.

Micropore
A small sized soil pore (approximately less than 30 microns in diameter) which is normally found within structural aggregates.

Microsite
A small part of the soil where the biological or chemical processes are different from the rest of the soil.

Mixotroph

Organisms that are capable of assimilating organic compounds as carbon sources, while using inorganic compounds as electron donors.

Mold
A group of saprobic or parasitic fungi causing a cottony growth on organic substances.

Monoclonal Antibody
Antibody produced from a single clone of cells, which has a uniform structure and specificity.

Monokaryon
Fungal hyphae where the compartments contain only nucleus.

Morphometric Characters
These are characteristics regarding the depth, dimension, sediment distribution, water currents etc.

Motility
The ability of a cell to move from one place to another.

Mucigel
Gelatinous material found on the surface of roots growing in normal soil.

Mucilage

Gelatinous secretions and exudates produced by plant roots and most micro-organisms.

Materials which are laid down on soil to protect it from rain, crusting, freezing etc. these materials could be sawdust, plastic, leaves etc.

Municipal Solid Waste
The total consumer and commercial waste generated in a certain confined and restricted geographic area.

Mycophagous
Organisms that eat fungi.

Mycovirus
Viruses that infect fungi.

Nanopore
Soil pore having dimensions in nanometers.

NAPL
A non-aqueous phase liquid which maybe lighter or denser than water.

Necrotrophic

A mechanism by which an organism produces lytic enzymes that kill and then breakdown host cells for its nutrition.

Nematode
Eukaryotes that are unsegmented, usually microscopic roundworm.

Neutralism
Lack of interaction between two organisms in the same habitat.

Niche
Functional role of an organism in a certain habitat.

Nictotinamide Adenine Dinucleotide (NAD+)
An important oxidized coenzyme that is a hydrogen and electron carrier in redox reactions.

Nicotinamide Adenine Dinucleotide Phosphate (NADP+)
An important oxidized coenzyme that acts as a hydrogen and electron carrier in various redox reactions.

Nitrate Reduction (biological)
The process of reduction of nitrate to simpler forms like ammonium by plant and micro-organisms.

Nitrification
Biological oxidation of ammonium to nitrite and nitrate.

Nitrifying Bacteria
Chemolithotrophs that can carry out the transformation from ammonia to nitrite or nitrate.

Nitrogen Cycle
The cycle where nitrogen is used by a living organism, then after the organism dies is restored to soil, followed by its final conversion to its original state of oxidation.

Nitrogenase
The enzyme required for biological nitrogen fixation.

Nodulin
Proteins produced in root hairs or nodules in response to rhizobial infection.

Nonpolar
A substance that is hydrophobic and does not easily dissolve in water.

Northern Blot
Hybridization of single stranded DNA or RNA to RNA fragments.

Nucleic Acid

A high molecular weight nucleotide polymer.

Nucleoid
The nuclear region of certain organisms like bacteria, which contains chromosomes, but which is not limited by a nuclear membrane.

Nucleophilic Compound
An electron donor in chemical reactions involving covalent catalysis in which the donated electrons bond with other chemical groups.

Oligonucleotide
A short nucleic acid chain, which is obtained from an organism or is synthesized chemically.

Oligotroph
A microorganism that has adapted itself to grow in environments that are low in nutrients.

Oospore
Thick walled spore formed in an oogonium by fungus like organisms like the phylum Oomycota.

Operon
Genes whose expression is controlled by a single operator.

Parasitism
Feeding by one organism on the cells of a second, normally larger organism, thus, harming the host.

Parasexual Cycle
A nuclear cycle wherein genes of haploid nuclei recombine without meiosis.

Particle Density
Density of particles present in soil.

Particle Size
Effective diameter of a particle measured by sedimentation or micrometric mathods.

Pasteurization
Process of using heat to kill or reduce the activity of micro-organisms in heat:sensitive materials.

Pathogen
An organism that is capable of causing an infection, or harming a host cell.

Pathogen Suppressive soil
Soil where a pathogen does not persist, either in its own survival or in its pathogenicity.

Pathogenicity

The ability of a parasite to infect or inflict damage on a host.

Peat
Unconsolidated soil material consisting mostly of undecomposed organic matter with excessive moisture content.

Pellicle
A rigid protein layer just below the cell membrane.

Peptidoglycan
Rigid cell wall layer seen in bacteria. It's also called murein.

Peribacteroid Membrane
A plant derived membrane which surrounds rhizobia in host cells of legume nodules.

Periplasmic space
The area between the cell membrane and cell wall in Gram negative bacteria.

Perithecium
Flask shaped ascocarp open at the tip.

Peritrichous Flagellation
Multiple flagella present all over the cell surface.

Permanent Wilting Point
The highest concentration of soil at which plants present in it, will irreversibly wilt when placed in a humid chamber.

Phosphobacterium
Bacteria that are good at dissolving insoluble inorganic phosphate that is present in soil.

Photoautotroph
Self-sufficient organisms that can generate energy from light and carbon dioxide.

Photoheterotroph
Organisms able to use light as source of energy and organic materials as carbon source.

Photophosphorylation
Synthesis of high energy phosphate bonds by the use of light as source of energy.

Phototaxis
Movement of an organism, or a part of it, towards light.

Phytoextraction
The use of plants or algae for removing contaminants from soil, sediments or water, and turning them into harvestable plant biomass.

Phycobilin
Water soluble pigment that is seen in cyanobacteria and is the light harvesting pigment for Photosystem II.

Pilus
Fimbria like substance present on fertile cells that deals with transfer of DNA during the process of conjugation.

Plaque
A localized area of lysis or cell inhibition which is caused due to virus infection.

Plasmogamy
Fusion of two cell contents, inclusive of the cytoplasm and nuclei.

Plate Count
Number of colonies formed on a solid culture medium, when uniformly inoculated with a known amount of soil.

Polar Flagellation
The presence of flagella at one or both ends.

Protoplast
A cell devoid of cell wall.

Pour Plate
The method of performing a plate count of micro-organisms.

Psychrotroph
An organism that is able to grow at zero degrees and above twenty degrees Celsius.

Pure Culture
A microorganism population of a single strain.

Radioimmunoassay
An immunological assay that makes use of radioactive antibodies or antigens to detect certain substances.

Reaction Center
A photosynthetic complex containing chlorophyll and other compounds.

Reannealing
The process seen on cooling, where two complementary strands of DNA hybridize back into a single strand.

Recalcitrant

Resistance of an organism to a microbial attack.

Recombination
Process by which genetic elements in two separate genomes are brought together in one unit. This is an important step in gene therapy.

Replication
Conversion of one double stranded DNA molecule into two identical double stranded DNA molecules.

Repression
Process by which an enzyme synthesis is suppressed due to the presence of certain external substance.

Reverse Transcription
Process of copying information from RNA to DNA.

Rhizobacteria
Bacteria that are found in roots, where they aggressively colonize.

Rhizobia
Bacteria capable of living symbiotically in leguminous plant roots, from where they receive energy and commonly fix molecular dinitrogen.

Rhizomorph
Mass of fungal hyphae that are organized in long, thick strands with a darkly pigmented outer rind that contains specialized tissues for absorption and water transport.

Rhizoplane
Plant root surface and strongly adhering soil particles.

Rhizosphere
The zone of soil immediately adjacent to plant roots in which the activity and type of micro-organisms present differ from that in the rest of the soil.

Rhizosphere Competence
Ability of an organism to colonize the rhizosphere.

Sanitization
Elimination of pathogenic or harmful organisms, including insect larvae, intestinal parasites and weed seeds.

Sclerotium
Modified fungal hyphae that form a compact and hard vegetative resting structure with a thick pigmented outer rind.

Secondary Metabolite
Product of intermediary metabolism released from a cell, for example, antibiotic.

Selective Medium
A medium that is biased in allowing only certain types of micro-organisms to grow.

Serial Dilution
Series of stepwise dilutions, normally done in sterile water, which is done to reduce microorganism populations to manageable numbers.

Serology
Study of reactions that take place between antigens and antibodies in vitro.

Sheath
Tubular structure that is found either around a chain of cells or around a bundle of filaments.

Siderochromes
The compounds that are synthesized by the micro-organisms themselves, which are responsible for iron uptake.

Siderophore
A metabolite that is formed by some micro-organisms, that forms a strong coordination compound with iron.

Slime Layer
A diffuse layer found immediately outside the cell wall in certain bacteria.

Slime Mold
Micro-organisms that are eukaryotic and which lack cell walls.

Solarization
A technique to control the growth of pathogens, wherein a plastic sheet is used to cover moistened soil in hot climates, thereby trapping the incoming radiation.

Specific Activity
Expressed as micromoles formed per unit time per milligram of protein, this is the amount of enzyme activity units per mass of protein.

Spermosphere
The area seen around a germinating seed, where there is increased microbiological activity.

Spread Plate
A technique for performing a plate count of micro-organisms.

Sterilization
The process whereby an object or surface is rendered free of any living micro-organisms.

Storage Polysaccharide
The energy reserves which are stored in a cell when there is excess of carbon available.

Strain
Population of cells, all of which arise from a single pure isolate.

Substrate
A base on which an organism is grown. They can also be the substances on which compounds and enzymes act.

Sulfur Cycle
The cycle wherein sulfur, the element is taken up by living organisms, then released upon the death of the organism, and then converted to its final state of oxidation.

Symbiosis
Two dissimilar organisms, living together. Their association maybe commensal or mutualistic.

Synergism
Association between two organisms that is mutually beneficial.

Syntrophy
Interaction between two or more populations that supply each other's nutritional needs.

Systemic
Something that involves the entire body and is not localized in the body.

Teichoic Acids
All wall, membrane or capsular polymers containing glycerophosphate or ribitol phosphate residues.

Telemorph
One of the stages of sexual reproduction, wherein cells are formed by meiosis and genetic recombination.

Temperate Virus
A virus that does not cause destruction and lysis of the cells of its host, but instead, its genome may replicate in sync with that of the host.

Terminal Electron Acceptor
The last acceptor of the electron, as it exits the electron transport chain.

Thermocline
That point in a lake, where there is a drastic drop in temperature with increase in depth.

Thermophile
An organism that grows best at temperatures around 45 and 80 degrees Celsius.

Ti plasmid
A conjugative tumor inducing plasmid that can transfer genes into plants. Seen in the bacterium Agrobacterium tunefaciens.

Toxin
A foreign substance present in the body, which is mostly generated by micro-organisms, that is capable of inflicting damage on the host cell.

Transduction
The process where host genetic information is transferred through an agent like a virus or a bacteriophage.

Transgenic
Genetically modified plants or organisms, which contain foreign genes, which have been inserted by means of recombinant DNA techniques.

Transposable Element
A genetic element that can be transposed from one site on a chromosome to another.

Transposon
Transposable element which, in addition to transposable genes, carries other genes.

Transposon Mutagenesis
A mutant phenotype is formed by inactivation of the host gene, which occurs due to the insertion of a transposon.

Tricarboxylic Acid Cycle
A series of metabolic reactions, by which pyruvate is oxidized to carbon dioxide.

Trophic Level
Describes the residence of nutrients in various organisms along a food chain ranging from the primary nutrient assimilating autotrophs to carnivorous animals.

Uronic Acid
A class of acidic compounds that contain both carboxylic and aldehydic groups and are oxidation products of sugars. They occur mainly in polysaccharides.

Vadose Zone
Unsaturated zone of soil which is above the groundwater, extending from the bottom of the capillary fringe to the soil surface.

Vector

An agent that can carry pathogens from one host to another. It can also denote a plasmid or virus used in genetic engineering to insert genes into a cell.

Vegetative Cell
A growing or actively feeding form of a cell, as against a spore.

Vesicles
Spherical structures formed intra:cellularly, by certain arbuscular mycorrhizal fungi.

Viable but Nonculturable
Living organisms that cannot be cultured on artificial media.

Viable Count
Measurement of the concentration of live cells in a microbial population.

Vibrio
Curved, rod-shaped bacteria that cause cholera, belonging to the genus Vibrio.

Virion
The virus particle and the virus nucleic acid surrounded by a protein coat.

Virulence
The degree of pathogenicity of a parasite.

Water Content
The amount of water contained in a material, which is expressed as the mass of water per unit mass of oven:dry material.

Water Retention Curve
A graph showing soil water content as a function of increasingly negative soil water potential.

White Rot Fungus
Fungus that attacks lignin, along with cellulose and hemicellulose, leading to marked lightening of the infected wood.

Wild Type
Strain of a microorganism that is isolated from nature. The native and original form of a gene or organism.

Winogradsky Column
A glass column that allows growth of micro-organisms under conditions similar to those found in nutrient rich water and sediment. This column contains an anerobic lower zone and an aerobic upper zone.

Woronin Body

A spherical structure found in fungi belonging to the phylum Ascomycota, which are associated with the simple pore in the septa separating the hyphal compartments.

Xenobiotic
A compound that is foreign to the biological systems.

Xerophile
An organism that is capable of growing at low water potentials, that is, in very dry habitats.

Zymogenous Flora
Refers to micro-organisms that respond rapidly by enzyme production and growth when simple organic substrates become available.

PHARMACOLOGY

Analgesic
Pain relief

Potentiates anesthesia

Narcotics

Medications given post op
Codeine (hydrocodone)

Meperidine (demerol)

Fentanyl (sublimaze)

Morphine (MS)

Inhalation Agents
Produces and maintains anesthesia

Usually liquid gasses

Puts you to sleep

Desflurane
Suprane

Requires the use of heated vaporizer

Sevoflurane
Ultrane

Odorless

Enflurane
Ethrane

Mild sweet odor

Halothane
Fluothane

Isoflurane
Forane

Pungent odor

Nitrous oxide
Only gas used in the or

Fruity odor

IV agents
Produces and maintains anesthesia

Dissociative agent
Ketamine (used for ages 2-10)

Most commonly used on mentally disabled patients

Also known as vitamin K (causes hallucinations in adults)

Opiates (narcotics)

Not typically given by ST
Morphine, meperidine (demerol), fentanyl (sublimaze), sufentanyl (Sufenta), Alfentanyl (Alfenta), Remifentanyl (Ultiva)

Benzodiazepines
Diazepam (Valium)

Midazolam (Vesed)- #1 relaxant- amnesia effect

Droperidol (Inapsine)

Nerve Conduction
Regional/ Local anesthesia

Mepivicaine
Carbocaine

Numb things

Bupivicaine
Marcaine

Numb Things

6-8 hours pain control

Lidocaine
Xylocaine

Fast acting

used in head and neck cases

usually mixed with epinephrine

18
Procaine
Novocaine

19
Cocaine
put on cotton balls

used to shrink the mucous membranes in the nose

Causes slight homeostasis

20
Tetracaine
Eye cases

21
Nerve Conduction Agonist
Enhances Anesthesia

22
Epinephrine
Vasoconstrictor

never used on fingers, toes, or penis

23
Wydase
not generally used

usually used in eye cases

24
Sedative/ hypnotic
Promotes sleep

reduces anxiety

25
Innovar
droperidol

Fentanyl

26
Phenobarbital
Rarely used

27
Anti Anxiety
reduce Anxiety

Potentiate Anesthesia

28
Diazepam

valium

Cataract surgery

colonoscopy

29
Vistaril
Hydroxizine Hydrochloride

30
Phenergan
Reduce Anxiety

31
Narcotic Antagonist
Neutralizer/ Reversal of Narcotics

32
Narcan
#1 drug given to drug addicts

Causes a hard reverse of the narcotic

33
Neuromuscular Block
Total muscle relaxation/paralyzes

34
Depolarizing
Causes fasciculations (twitching)

Succinylcholine

Anectine

Syncurine

35
Non-Depolarizing
No Twitches

Curare- Used by Indians to poison arrows

Atracurium-Tracium

36
Pancuronium
Pavulon

37
Vercuronium
Norcuron

38
Mivicron
Non-Depolarizing

39

Zemuron
Non-Depolarizing

40

Neuromuscular Antagonist
Reverses Muscle Relaxation

Protigmine-Neostigmine

Antagonize Non- depolarizing

41

Anti-Inflammatories
Reduces inflammation- typically used in Ortho cases or noids

42

Non Steroidal
NSAID

Ketaloric-Toradol

Basically Tylenol on Steroids

43

Steroidal
Hydrocortisone- Solu-Cortef

Methylprednisone-Solu-medrol

Dexamethasone-Decadron

Betamethasone- Celestone

44

Methylprednisone
Soul-medrol

Used for back pain, knee surgery

Usually mixed with a local

45

Dexamethasone
Decadron

Used on tonsil surgery

Usually given at the start of the case 8-10 mg

46

Antimuscarinic
Blocks secretions

Prevents spasms

Inhibits parasymphetic responses

IE: Atropine, Robinal

47
Anticonvulsant
Prevents Siezures

IE: Magnesium Sulfate

48
Enzymes
Muscle Relaxant for MH

Dantrolene- Dantrium

Pre mix before giving.... comes in a powder

49
Electrolyte Replacement
Combat metabolic acidosis

Sodium Bicarbonate (usually during codes)

50
Diuretic
Heart Issues/Edema

51
Lasix
#1 diuretic

Increases urine output

52
Mannitol
Reduces edema

Crain cases

Big cases

Swelling 2 degrees ICP

53
Histamine2 (H2)
Decreases gastric activity and volume

High BMI always get this

54
Tagamet
Cimetadine

55
Zantec
Ranitidine

56
Hormone

Supplement/Replacement

Glycogen
Smooth Muscle relaxant

Insulin
Humulin

Oxytocic
Contracts Uterus

Usually used for D&C cases or c-section

IE: Pitocin-Oxytocin

Bronchodilator
Expands Lumen of Upper Reps. Tract

Asthma Attack

Given: Aminophyline

Ephedrine- only given if they are about to faint

Stains
Identify Abnormal Tissue (Usually Iodine Based)

Discolors

Lugol's solution or Schiller's solution

White vinegar can be used (This stains the bad tissue) Used in Cervix biopsies

Dyes
Enhances visualization

Mark Incision lines

Methylene Blue- Used in breast reductions, varicose veins, and infertility determinations

Indigo Carmine- Used in breast reductions, varicose veins, and infertility determinations

Gentain Violet

Contrast Media
Enhances X-Rays

Used to find stones or strictures

Important to get all air out of the syringe before injection

Examples of Contrast Media
Hypague

Reno-M-30

Reno-M-60

Grafin

Hyskon

Omnipaque

Hemostatic Agents
Gelatin Sponges

Collagen

Cellulose

Thrombin

Protamine-Heparin Reversal (Open Heart)

Anticoagulant
Prevents Clotting

Heparin- Open Heart

Warfin- Coumadin- This is oral, not typically given in OR usually given after Total Knee arthroscopy, valves, and stents

Coagulation Agents
Forms Clots

Calcium Gluconate

Vitamin K

Vasodilator
Dilates Peripheral Blood Vessels

Raises BP

Vasopressin

Aramine

Levophed- If you have to use this its not a good sign

Coronary Artery Dilator

Increases Blood Flow to heart

Nitro- not given in the OR

Antihypertensive
Reduces BP

Nitropress

Niprine

Procardia

Antiarrythmic
Corrects cardiac arrythmias

1) Lidocaine

2) Calcium Chloride (Myocardial Stimulator)

3) Potassium Chloride

Cardiac Glycoside
Increase Cardiac Output

Digoxin

IV Solutions
Provides hydration, enhances renal function, Route of Admin, provides calories (D5W), provides nutrition, plasma expander (used in increase blood loss), Artificial Plasma, balanced solution similar to plasma

Irrigation Solutions
Normal Saline

Sterile Distilled Water

BSS- Balanced Salt Solution (used in eye cases)

Miotic
Constricts Pupils

Acetylcholine (usually given post op)

Pilocarpine

Mydriatic
Dilates Pupils

Pre-op for cataract surgery

Cyclogyn

Before Surgery

Adrenergic
Stimulates Nerve Fibers

Epinephrine

Adrenaline

Antibiotic
Antibacterial

Bacitracin

Ancef

Kanamycin- kantrex

Neomycin

Vancomycin- used for bigger cases

Tobradex- antibiotic and antiinflammatory

Antiemetic
Reduce Nausea and Vomiting

Droperidol- inapsine

Reglan

Antihistamine
Counteracts Allergic Reactions

Benadryl

Neuroleptanesthesia
When neuroleptanalgesia is reinforced with an inhalation or IV anesthetic

Perfect anesthesia

TESTS AND ANSWERS

Which of the following is the wound classification for a bronchoscopy?

A. Clean

B. Contaminated

C. Dirty and Infected

D. Clean-contaminated

D. Clean-contaminated

The enzyme used to soften the zonules of the lens before cataract surgery is:

A. Atropine Sulfate

B. Alpha-chymotrypsin

C. Acetylcholine chloride

D. Pilocarpine hydrochloride

B. Alpha-chymotrypsin

How should the stretcher be oriented when necessary to use an elevator to transport a patient to the OR?

A. Place stretcher sideways in elevator

B. Enter head first, exit feet first

C. Position in elevator is irrelevant

D. Enter feet first, exit head first

B. Enter head first, exit feet first

Which of the following is a curved, transverse incision across the lower abdomen frequently used in gynecological surgery?

A. Midline

B. Paramedian

C. McBurney's

D. Pfannenstiel

D. Pfannenstiel

When perforated metal trays are placed on the shelves of the steam sterilizing cart, they should be positioned:

A. Flat

B. Upside Down

C. Vertical

D. Angled

A. Flat

Hyperkalemia is a high concentration of:

A. Calcium

B. Nitrogen

C. Potassium

D. Albumin

C. Potassium

Which of the following tissues are cut using curved Mayo scissors?

A. Fascia

B. Periosteum

C. Dura mater

D. Arterial wall

A. Fascia

Which laser beam can travel through clear tissues without heating them?

A. Argon

B. Excimer

C. Carbon dioxide

D. Neodymium: YAG

A. Argon

Permission for treatment given with full knowledge of the risks is a/an:
A. Tort
B. Malpractice
C. Personal liability
D. Informed consent

D. Informed consent

Which portion of the stomach surrounds the lower esophageal sphincter?
A. Cardia
B. Fundus
C. Pylorus
D. Antrum

A. Cardia

Low level disinfectants kill most microbes, but do not destroy:
A. Viruses
B. Bacteria
C. Fungi
D. Spores

D. Spores

Syndactyly refers to:
A. Celft palate
B. Webbed fingers
C. Fused tarsals
D. Torn ligaments

B. Webbed fingers

The surgical pack utilized to create the sterile field should be opened on the:
A. Stretcher
B. OR table
C. Backtable
D. Mayo stand

C. Backtable

The islets of Langerhans secrete:
A. Bile
B. Insulin
C. Intrinsic factor
D. Inhibiting hormones

B. Insulin

What type of procedure would involve the removal of teeth?
A. Cleft palate repair
B. Arch bar application
C. Extractions
D. Implants

C. Extractions

Which organism is normal resident flora of the intestinal tract?
A. Escherichia coli
B. Staphylococcus aureus
C. Psudomonas aeruginosa
D. Clostridium tetani

A. Escherichia coli

Where should the first scrub surgical technologist stand when handing towels to the surgeon to square off an incision site?

A. Opposite side from surgeon

B. Same side as surgeon

C. Foot of OR table

D. Head of OR table

B. Same side as surgeon

A properly performed surgical scrub renders the skin:

A. Sterile

B. Disinfected

C. Surgically clean

D. Moistened anddehydrated

C. Surgically clean

Through which of the following do the common bile duct and the pancreatic duct empty?

A. Ampulla of Vater

B. Duct of Santorini

C. Wirsung's duct

D. Sphincter of Oddi

A. Ampulla of Vater

Which of the following identifiers must be verified by the patient or their ID bracelet prior to transporting a patient to the OR?

A. Name, social security #, physician

B. Name, medical record #, allergies

C. Name, date of birth, diagnosis

D. Name, date of birth, physician

D. Name, date of birth, physician

What are spiral-shaped bacteria called?
A. Cocci
B. Bacilli
C. Sprilli
D. Diplococci

C. Spirilli

The primary function of the gallbladder is to:
A. Store bile
B. Produce bile
C. Emulsify fats
D. Metabolize fats

A. Store bile

Which of the following is a non-sterile member of the surgical team?
A. Surgeon
B. Circulator
C. Surgical assistant
D. Surgical technologist

B. Circulator

Which of the following is not a benefit of using surface-mounted sliding doors for access to the operating room?
A. Uses less space for opening
B. Aid in controlling temperature
C. Eliminate air turbulence
D. Provides for thorough cleaning

D. Provides for thorough cleaning

What are three factors for reducing ionizing radiation exposure?

A. Type of procedure, equipment, radiation dose

B. Exposure, frequency, concentration

C. Time, shielding, distance

D. Site, age, gender

C. Time, shielding, distance

Which is the first part of the small intestine?

A. Duodenum

B. Jejunum

C. Ileum

D. Cecum

A. Duodenum

What is the surgical position frequently used for patients undergoing kidney surgery?

A. Prone

B. Lateral

C. Supine

D. Lithotomy

B. Lateral

How are rickettsiae transmitted?

A. Arthropod bites

B. Physical contact

C. Blood exposure

D. Airborne organisms

A. Arthropod bites

Which of the following is an examination of the cervix using a binocular microscope?
A. Colposcopy
B. Laparoscopy
C. Urethroscopy
D. Hysteroscopy

A. Colposcopy

Compression of the heart from excessive fluid or blood buildup is called:
A. Tamponade
B. Pericarditis
C. Infarction
D. Cardiomyopathy

A. Tamponade

Which surgical team member determines when the patient can be transported from the OR to the PACU?
A. Anesthesia provider
B. Circulator
C. Surgeon
D. Surgical technologist

A. Anesthesia provider

Which suffix means surgical puncture to remove fluid?
A. -dynia
B. -tomy

C. -lysis

D. –centesis

D. -centesis

To which portion of the colon is the appendix attached?

A. Ascending

B. Descending

C. Cecum

D. Sigmoid

C. Cecum

Which laboratory test determines bacterial identification?

A. Gram stain

B. Manual count

C. Prothrombin time

D. Gel electrophoresis

A. Gram stain

Medication used to dilate the pupil is called:

A. Miotics

B. Myopics

C. Mydriatics

D. Muscarinics

C. Mydriatics

Which of the following drapes is non-fenestrated?

A. Laparotomy

B. U-drape

C. Transverse

D. Craniotomy

B. U-drape

Under what circumstances would it be appropriate to remove a patient's identification bracelet?

A. During insertion of an IV catheter

B. Never until patient is discharged from facility

C. Postoperatively when taken to the nursing unit

D. When patient is awake and alert and can verbally identify self

B. Never until patient is discharged from facility

What is the position most commonly used for mitral valve replacement?

A. Prone

B. Sims

C. Supine

D. Kraske

C. Supine

Which laser is used during a vitrectomy?

A. Carbon dioxide

B. Nd:YAG

C. Excimer

D. Argon

D. Argon

Which of the following monitors provides positive assurance of sterility?

A. Clerical

B. Mechanical

C. Biological

D. Chemical

C. Biological

The apron-like structure attached to the greater curvature of the stomach is the:

A. Omentum

B. Mesentery

C. Ligamentum

D. Peritoneum

A. Omentum

Which microbes live without oxygen?

A. Aerobes

B. Anaerobes

C. Capnophiles

D. Microaerophiles

B. Anaerobes

Which of the following is an abnormal tract between two epithelium-lined surfaces that is open at both ends?

A. Epitheliazation

B. Fistula

C. Herniation

D. Sinus

B. Fistula

What is the action of antagonist drugs?
A. Inhibit of the clotting process
B. Achieve neuroleptanesthesia
C. Increase the effects of opiates
D. Counteract the action of another drug

D. Counteract the action of another drug

Which of the following directional terms describes the type of skin prep of an entire extremity?
A. Spiral
B. Horizontal
C. Longitudinal
D. Circumferential

D. Circumferential

What organs are excised if an ovarian tumor is malignant?
A. Bilateral ovaries only
B. Bilateral fallopian tubes and ovaries, uterus
C. Unilateral involved ovary and fallopian tube
D. Unilateral involved ovary and fallopian tube, uterus

B. Bilateral fallopian tubes and ovaries, uterus

Which term refers to an abnormal thoracic curve of the spin referred to as "hunchback"?
A. Lordosis
B. Scoliosis
C. Kyposis
D. Alkalosis

C. Kyphosis

What is the medical term for a bunion?

A. Talipes valgus

B. Hallux valgus

C. Hallux varus

D. Talipes varus

B. Hallux valgus

What incision is also known as a lower oblique?

A. Ingiunal

B. Paramedian

C. Infraumbilical

D. Thoracoabdominal

A. Ingiunal

The small intestine attaches to the posterior abdominal wall by the:

A. Mesentery

B. Peritoneum

C. Falciform ligament

D. Lesser omentum

A. Mesentery

What is the term for a relationship in which two organisms occupy the same area and one organism benefits while the other is unharmed?

A. Commensialism

B. Neutralism

C. Mutualism

D. Parasitism

A. Commensalism

A topical steroid used to reduce inflammation after eye surgery is:

A. Deop-Medrol

B. Miochol

C. Healon

D. Wydase

A. Depo-Medrol

How is the surgical informed consent signed if an adult patient is illiterate?

A. Authorized individual signs patient's name

B. Patient marks with an "X" and witness verifies

C. RN and surgeon sign that patient gave consent

D. Surgeon and Risk Manager sign consent

B. Patient marks with an "X" and witness verifies

What direction should the stretcher be oriented when transporting a patient to the OR department?

A. Feet first, side rails up

B. Feet first, side rails down

C. Head first, side rails up

D. Head first, side rails down

A. Feet first, side rails up

Which of the following routine preoperative laboratory studies would be ordered for premenopausal women with no history of hysterectomy?

A. HCG

B. HBV

C. HIV

D. HDL

A. HCG

Which portion of the surgical gown is considered non-sterile?
A. Outside closure ties
B. Two inches below neckline to table level
C. Upper arms, neckline and axillary region
D. Sleeves; two inches above the elbows to the cuffs

C. Upper arms, neckline and axillary region

What is the name of the urinary catheter with a small, curved tapered tip used on patients with urethral strictures?
A. Iglesias
B. Coude
C. Pigtail
D. Bonanno

B. Coude

What is the surgical position commonly used for thyroid and gallbladder surgery?
A. Supine
B. Fowler's
C. Reverse Trendelenburg
D. Lateral Kidney

C. Reverse Trendelenburg

A congenital defect in which the fetal blood vessel between the pulmonary artery and aorta does not close is:
A. Coarctation of the aorta
B. Patent ductus arteriosus
C. Tetralogy of Fallot
D. Ventricular septal defect

D. Ventricular septal defect

Which of the following is a commonly used preservative for tissue specimens?
A. Saline
B. Formalin
C. Ethyl alcohol
D. Lugol's solution

B. Formalin

What is the first step taken for an incorrect sponge count?
A. Notify surgeon
B. X-ray patient
C. Repeat count
D. Complete incident report

A. Notify surgeon

The mumps may be diagnosed by finding inflammation in which of the following glands?
A. Sublingual
B. Thyroid
C. Parotid
D. Submandibular

B. Thyroid

What institutional document is completed when an adverse or unusual event takes place in the OR that may have legal consequences for the staff or patient?
A. Incident report
B. Operative record
C. Deposition report
D. Advance directive

A. Incident report

For which procedure would Trendelenburg position provide optimal visualization?

A. Cholecystectomy

B. Hysterectomy

C. Thyroidectomy

D. Acromioplasty

B. Hysterectomy

Which of the following is a nonadherent dressing?

A. Kling

B. Adaptic

C. Collodion

D. Elastoplast

B. Adaptic

Which of the following is a fenestrated drape?

A. Incise

B. U-drape

C. Aperture

D. Half-sheet

C. Aperture

Which of the following terms describes a hernia that occurs within Hesselbach's triangle?

A. Direct

B. Indirect

C. Femoral

D. Hiatal

A. Direct

Which of the following incision is oblique?

A. Epigastric

B. Kocher

C. Paramedian

D. Pfannenstiel

B. Kocher

Which of the following dilators are used in the common duct?

A. Pratt

B. Van Buren

C. Bakes

D. Hegar

C. Bakes

Which of the following is a mechanical method of hemostasis?

A. Laser

B. Ligature

C. Thrombin

D. Electrosurgery

B. Ligature

The organ that is connected by a duct to the duodenum is the:

A. Pancreas

B. Gallbladder

C. Stomach

D. Liver

A. Pancreas

A brain tumor causing alteration of muscle tone, voluntary muscle coordination, gait and balance would likely be located in the:

A. Diencephalon

B. Cerebellum

C. Medulla

D. Pons

B. Cerebellum

What is the term for a relationship that benefits one organism at the expense of another?

A. Commensalism

B. Neutralism

C. Mutualism

D. Parasitism

D. Parasitism

What type of disease is characterized by rapid onset and a rapid recovery?

A. Acute

B. Chronic

C. Primary

D. Asymptomatic

A. Acute

Which organelle is responsible for the production of energy?

A. Lysosomes

B. Mitochondria

C. Golgi complex

D. Endoplasmic reticulum

B. Mitochondria

What type of anesthesia is a combination of inhalation and intravenous drugs?
A. Spinal
B. Sedation
C. Regional
D. Balanced

D. Balanced

Who is ultimately responsible for obtaining the surgical informed consent?
A. Guardian
B. Patient
C. Surgeon
D. Nurse

C. Surgeon

What position is most commonly used for neurosurgical procedures?
A. Supine
B. Semi-Fowler's
C. Trendelenburg
D. Lithotomy

A. Supine

The outer layer of the intestine is the:
A. Mucosa
B. Serosa
C. Muscularis
D. Submucosa

B. Serosa

Which of the following solutions should be used to prep the donor site for split-thickness skin graft?
A. Iodophor
B. Avagard
C. Chlorhexidine
D. Merthiolate

C. Chlorhexidine

What type of drape would be used for a flank procedure?
A. Transverse
B. Extremity
C. Aperture
D. Perineal

A. Transverse

Where should the safety strap be placed on a patient who is in the supine position?
A. Below the knees
B. Across the waist
C. Over the thighs
D. Across the abdomen

C. Over the thighs

Which surgical procedure is performed to correct an abnormality in which the urethral meatus is situation on the superior aspect of the penis?
A. Hypospadias repair
B. Epispadias repair

C. Meatotomy

D. Ureteroneocystostomy

B. Epispadias repair

Which thermal method of hemostasis utilizes intense, focused light?

A. Laser

B. Bipolar

C. Harmonic

D. Monopolar

A. Laser

What is the most common cause of intracerebral hemorrhage?

A. Hypotension

B. Hypertension

C. Meningioma

D. Meningitis

B. Hypertension

The larynx is located between the:

A. Pharynx and trachea

B. Nasal cavity and pharynx

C. Trachea and bronchi

D. Nasal and oral cavities

A. Pharynx and trachea

The most common cause of retinal detachment is:

A. Aging

B. Trauma

C. Glaucoma

D. Inflammation

B. Trauma

What postoperative complication is associated with total hip arthroplasty?

A. Compartment syndrome

B. Upper extremity weakness

C. Urinary incontinence

D. Pulmonary embolism

D. Pulmonary embolism

Which of the following is a type of passive drain?

A. Penrose

B. Hemovac

C. Pleur-evac

D. Jackson-Pratt

A. Penrose

The vocal cords are located in the:

A. Pharynx

B. Larynx

C. Trachea

D. Bronchus

B. Larynx

What type of acquired immunity is a vaccination?

A. Artificial passive

B. Artificial active

C. Natural passive

D. Natural active

B. Artificial active

When would the anesthesia provider request cricoid pressure?

A. Bier block

B. Epidural injection

C. Endotracheal intubation

D. Endotracheal extubation

C. Endotracheal intubation

Which instrument would be used during a keratoplasty to remove the cornea?

A. Trephine

B. Westcott

C. Oculotome

D. Phacoemulsifier

A. Trephine

What is the required minimum number of individuals to transfer an incapacitated patient from the OR table to the stretcher?

A. 3

B. 4

C. 5

D. 6

B. 4

Which of the following regulations states that blood and body fluids should be considered infectious?

A. Body Substance Isolation Rules

B. Medical Device Safety Act

C. Postexposure Prophylaxis

D. Standard Precautions

D. Standard Precautions

Which of the following is a major source of distress for toddler and preschool age patients being transported to the operating room?

A. Room temperature change

B. Lack of communication

C. Fear of anesthesia

D. Separation anxiety

D. Separation anxiety

Which structure has oral, nasal, and laryngeal divisions?

A. Esophagus

B. Trachea

C. Pharynx

D. Glottis

C. Pharynx

Otoplasty is performed to correct a congenital deformity of which structure?

A. Mouth

B. Nose

C. Ear

D. Eye

C. Ear

An injury a patient sustains as a result of the care given by a healthcare professional is called:

A. Iatrogenic

B. Liability

C. Battery

D. Tort

A. Iatrogenic

The highly vascular layer of the eye that absorbs light rays and nourishes the retina is the:

A. Sclera

B. Iris

C. Choroid

D. Macula

C. Choroid

According to Maslow's hierarchy of needs, which of the following is the patient satisfying when he/she trusts the surgical team's abilities?

A. Physiological

B. Belonging

C. Esteem

D. Safety

D. Safety

Whch aneurysm usually develops between the renal and iliac arteries?

A. Ascending thoracic

B. Aortic arch

C. Descending thoracic

D. Abdominal aortic

D. Abdominal aortic

The agent used to flush an artery to prevent clotting is:
A. Heparin
B. Thrombin
C. Protamine Sulfate
D. Ringer's Lactate

A. Heparin

What is the next step for reattachment of a severed digit after debridement?
A. Vessel reanastomosis
B. Nerve reanastomosis
C. Bone-to-bone fixation
D. Tendon-to-tendon fixation

C. Bone-to-bone fixation

What type of skin graft includes the epidermis and all of the dermis?
A. Composite
B. Split-thickness
C. Pedicle
D. Full-thickness

D. Full-thickness

Which muscle type is striated and voluntary?
A. Visceral
B. Heart
C. Skeletal
D. Cardiac

C. Skeletal

Which of the following terms refers to absence of the external ear?

A. Microtia

B. Anophthalmia

C. Cheiloschisis

D. Extrosyndactyly

A. Microtia

What is the recommended maximum time limit for a tourniquet to remain inflated on an adult lower extremity?

A. 30 minutes

B. 60 minutes

C. 1 1/2 hours

D. 2 1/2 hours

C. 1 1/2 hours

Which organism causes gas gangrene?

A. Clostridium perfringens

B. Clostridium botulinum

C. Staphylococcus aureus

D. Staphylococcus epidermidis

A. clostridium perfingens

Chest rolls should span the distance bilaterally between which two anatomical structures?

A. Nipple to umbilicus

B. Iliac crest to iliac crest

C. Scapula to gluteus maximus

D. Acromioclavicular joint to iliac crest

D. Acromioclavicular joint to iliac crest

Which ossicle of the middle ear covers the oval window?

A. Malleus

B. Incus

C. Stapes

D. Utricle

C. Stapes

What is another name for the Kraske position?

A. Dorsal recumbent

B. Jackknife

C. Trendelenburg

D. Beach chair

B. Jackknife

What type of sponge is tightly rolled cotton tape used by surgeons for blunt dissection?

A. Raytec

B. Kitner

C. Weck-Cel

D. Cottonoid

B. Kitner

Which of these instruments would be used during a keratoplasty?

A. Kilner hook

B. Bowman probe

C. Kerrison rongeur

D. Cottingham punch

D. Cottingham punch

A partially dislocated joint is called:

A. Sublaxation

B. Malrotation

C. Avulsion

D. Malunion

A. Sublaxation

What condition is characterized by build-up of fatty deposits such as cholesterol?

A. Embolism

B. Thrombosis

C. Arteriospasm

D. Atherosclerosis

D. Atherosclerosis

Plaster rolls for casting should be submerged in which of the following?

A. Lukewarm saline

B. Lukewarm water

C. Cold saline

D. Cold water

B. Lukewarm water

The avascular, clear portion of he eye covering the iris is the:

A. Cornea

B. Sclera

C. Pupil

D. Conjunctiva

A. Cornea

How often should surgical masks be changed?

A. After lunch

B. Twice-a-day

C. After each case

D. Every two hours

C. After each case

Which term describes a rod-shaped microorganism?

A. Coccus

B. Bacillus

C. Sprillum

D. Helical

B. Bacillus

When using the warm cycle on the EtO sterilizer, what is the minimum sterilization termperature in Fahrenheit?

A. 55

B. 65

C. 75

D. 85

D. 85

Which of the following actions would be a violation of aseptic technique?

A. Cuffing the hands within the drape

B. Sterile person reaching over sterile surface

C. Repositioning penetrating towel clip

D. Sterile surgical members passing face-to-face

C. Repositioning penetrating towel clip

Which legal principle applies when the patient is given the wrong dose of the local anesthetic?
A. Res ipsa loquitor
B. Respondeat superior
C. Bona fide
D. Assualt

A. Res ipsa loquitor

The space between the vocal cords s called the:
A. Epiglottis
B. Glottis
C. Vocal fold
D. Cricoid cartilage

B. Glottis

Which bacteria could be found in a penetrating wound caused by a rusty nail?
A. Treponema pallidum
B. Bacillus anthracis
C. Clostridium tetani
D. Helicobacter pylori

C. Clostridium tetani

Which of the following retractors is used for spinal nerve roots?
A. Taylor
B. Love
C. Cushing
D. Meyerding

B. Love

What is another name for the electrosurgical unit's patient return electrode?

A. Cautery

B. Generator

C. Foot pedal

D. Grounding pad

D. Grounding pad

What size of Foley catheter is commonly used for adults?

A. 8 Fr

B. 12 Fr

C. 16 Fr

D. 24 Fr

C. 16 Fr

Which of the following tumors is typically benign, encapsulated, and arises from tissue covering the central nervous system structures?

A. Meningioma

B. Astrocytoma

C. Schwannoma

D. Oligodendroglioma

A. Meningioma

The fibrous white layer that gives the eye its shape is the:

A. Iris

B. Cornea

C. Sclera

D. Choroid

C. Sclera

What is the term for thread-like appendages that provide bacteria with motion?

A. Flagella

B. Fimbriae

C. Mesosomes

D. Mitochondria

A. Flagella

What surgical position provides optimal visualization of the lower abdomen or pelvis?

A. Fowler's

B. Reverse Trendelenburg

C. Trendelenburg

D. Kraske

C. Trendelenburg

How many hours must an item submerse in glutaraldehyde to sterilize?

A. 7

B. 8

C. 9

D. 10

D. 10

When a patient's blood pressure is 135/81, 135 refers to:

A. Diastolic

B. Systolic

C. Pedal pulse

D. Apical pressure

B. Systolic

A term referring to a waxy secretion in the external ear canal is:

A. Mucous

B. Sputum

C. Cerumen

D. Perilymph

C. Cerumen

Which of the following is an ossicle of the middle ear?

A. Pinna

B. Incus

C. Labyrinth

D. Vestibule

B. Incus

What is the term for the process of removing blood from an extremity prior to inflating the pneumatic tourniquet?

A. Exsanguination

B. Extravasation

C. Evisceration

D. Evacuation

A. Exsanguination

Which of the following may require probing and dilating in pediatric patients with upper respiratory infections?

A. Sinus cavities

B. Eustachian tube

C. Nasolacrimal duct

D. Tympanic membrane

C. Nasolacrimal duct

Which surgical team member is responsible for setting up the sterile field?
A. Surgical first assistant
B. Surgical technologist
C. Circulating nurse
D. Surgeon

B. Surgical technologist

In what circumstances would cell-saver transfusion be contraindicated?
A. Anemica patients
B. Diabetic patients
C. Cancer procedures
D. Orthopedic procedures

C. Cancer procedures

Use of an intraluminal (circular) stapler (EEA) would be indicated for which of the following surgical procedures?
A. Pancreatectomy
B. Cholecystectomy
C. Polypectomy
D. Sigmoidectomy

D. Sigmoidectomy

Satinsky, Herrick, and Mayo clamps may be specifically used on which of the following structures?
A. Kidney pedicle
B. Seminal vesicle

C. Bladder neck

D. Prostate gland

A. Kidney pedicle

The nasal cavity is divided into two portions by the:

A. Ethmoid

B. Septum

C. Vomer

D. Sphenoid

B. Septum

Which of the following is used by the surgeon to intermittently remove prostatic tissue fragments during a TURP?

A. Randall froceps

B. Wire snare

C. Ellik evacuator

D. Poole suction

C. Ellik evacuator

Which type of hematoma is a result of torn bridging meningeal veins?

A. Subdural

B. Epidural

C. Intracerebral

D. Intraventricular

A. Subdural

In addition to temperature, time and moisture, what is the fourth factor that determines the outcome of the steam sterilization process?

A. Concentration

B. Aeration

C. Weight

D. Pressure

D. Pressure

The Bowie-Dick test is performed:

A. Hourly

B. Daily

C. Weekly

D. Monthly

B. Daily

The spiral, conical structure of the inner ear is the:

A. Cochela

B. Stapes

C. Vestibule

D. Labyrinth

A. Cochlea

What is the name of the condition in which a loop of bowel herniates into the Douglas's cul-de-sac?

A. Cystocele

B. Rectocele

C. Enterocele

D. Omphalocele

C. Entereocle

Which of these conditions is characterized by a fleshy encroachment of conjunctiva onto the cornea?

A. Chalazion

B. Pterygium

C. Strabismus

D. Ecchymosis

B. Pterygium

Which procedure would be listed in the OR schedule for a patient undergoing surgical treatment of uterine fibroids?

A. Pelvic exenteration

B. Cervical cerclage

C. Colporrhaphy

D. Myomoectomy

D. Myomectomy

Where is a Baker's cyst located?

A. Olecranon process

B. Greater tubercle

C. Popliteal fossa

D. Carpal tunnel

C. Popliteal fossa

Which of the following is a method of high-level disinfection?

A. Peracetic acid for 30 minutes

B. 2 % glutaraldehyde for 20 minutes

C. Steam under pressure for 10 minutes

D. Hydrogen peroxide gas plasma for 75 minutes

B. 2 % glutaradehyde for 20 minutes

Another name for the tympanic membrane is the:
A. Ear tube
B. Ear canal
C. Earlobe
D. Eardrum

D. Eardrum

What is the burn degree classification that involves the epidermis and subcutaneous tissue?
A. First
B. Second
C. Third
D. Fourth

C. Third

Which portion of the ear is affected by Meniere's syndrome?
A. Inner
B. Middle
C. Eustachian tube
D. Auditory ossicles

A. Inner

The cartilaginous nasal septum is anterior to which bone?
A. Hyoid
B. Vomer
C. Mandible
D. Palatine

B. Vomer

The most reliable method for determining the efficiency of moist heat sterilizers is the controlled use of biological indicators containing the organism:

A. Bacillus sterothermophilus
B. Clostridium tetani
C. Bordetella pertussis
D. Corynebacterium diphtheria

A. Bacillus stearothermophilus

Which neurosurgical pathaology would a myelogram diagnose?

A. Subdural hematoma
B. Creutzfeldt-Jakob
C. Spinal stenosis
D. Myelomeningocele

C. Spinal stenosis

Which of the following terms means a prolapsed bladder causing a bulge in the anterior vaginal wall?

A. Rectocele
B. Cystocele
C. Enterocele
D. Herniation

B. Cystocele

How many hours must the steam sterilization biological indicator incubate?

A. 6
B. 12
C. 18
D. 24

D. 24

The nasal sinus located between the nose and the orbits is the:

A. Frontal

B. Sphenoid

C. Ethmoid

D. Maxillary

C. Ethmoid

What is the definition of otosclerosis?

A. Earache

B. Tinnitus

C. Tearing of tympanic membrane

D. Bony overgrowth of stapes

D. Bony overgrowth of stapes

Which of the following terms describes a fracture in which the bone penetrates the skin?

A. Comminuted

B. Compound

C. Simple

D. Closed

B. Compound

For which of the following procedures would a McBurney incision be indicated?

A. Apendectomy

B. Cholecystectomy

C. Herniorrhaphy

D. Gastrectomy

A. Appendectomy

What degrees Celsius is the steam sterilization biological indicator incubated?

A. 43-48

B. 49-54

C. 55-60

D. 61-66

C. 55-60

What is the medical term for removal of the uterus?

A. Salpingectomy

B. Oophorectomy

C. Myomectomy

D. Hysterectomy

D. Hysterectomy

Which of the following methods removes small organic particles and soil from the box locks and ratchets of instruments?

A. Ultrasonic washer

B. Manual cleaning

C. Washer-sterilizer

D. Enzymatic soak

A. Ultrasonic washer

What is the medical term for nosebleed?

A. Rhinitis

B. Sinusitis

C. Epistaxis

D. Hemoptysis

C. Epistaxis

What is the proper method for preparing a Frazier suction tip for steam sterilization?

A. Lumen is dry

B. Distilled water in lumen

C. Stylet is left inside lumen

D. Disinfectant solution in lumen

B. Distilled water in lumen

Which of the following is a telescoping of the intestines in neonates requiring immediate surgical intervention?

A. Intussusception

B. Pyloric stenosis

C. Tetralogy of Fallot

D. Omphalocele

A. Intussusception

The minimum Fahrenheit temperature for sterilization to occur in a prevacuum steam sterilizer is:

A. 249-255

B. 256-262

C. 263-269

D. 270-276

D. 270-276

Wat is the name of the procedure for the excision of the tunica vaginalis?

A. Spermatocelectomy

B. Orhiectomy

C. Hydrocelectomy

D. Vasectomy

C. Hydrocelectomy

What is the minimum number of minutes to sterilize unwrapped metal instruments with lumens in the gravity displacement sterilizer at 270 degrees farhenheit?

A. 5
B. 10
C. 15
D. 20

B. 10

A lumbar puncture removes cerebral spinal fluid from

a. The subarachnoid space
b. The epidural space
c. The lateral ventricle of the brain
d. The space between C-1 and C-2

A. The subarachnoid space

Cold, clammy skin may be a symptom of:

a. Hypothermia
b. Hyperthermia
c. Hypertension
d. Shock

D. Shock

Which of the following is an atraumatic clamp?

a. Kocher
b. Allis

c. Heaney

d. Babcock

D. Babcock

The ophthalmic medication which causes pupils to constrict is:

a. Mydriatic

b. Miotic

c. Cycloplegic

d. Corticosteroid

B. Miotic

A fracture of the frontal process of the maxilla. Nasal bones and orbital floor would be classified as a(n):

a. Le Fort I

b. Le Fort II

c. Le Fort III

d. Malar Fracture

B. Le Fort II

Crushing urinary stones is commonly referred to as:

a. Lithotripsy

b. Nephrolithtomy

c. KUB

d. TURL

a. Lithotripsy

A procedure performed to correct urinary incontinence is:

a. Werheim

b. Cerclage

C. Mashall-Marchetti

D. D & E

c. Mashall-Marchetti

The CBD joins the duodenum at this juncture:

a. Ampulla of Vater

b. Sphincter of Oddi

c. Duct of Wirsung

D. Biliary duct

a. Ampulla of Vater

The active electrode in a Monopolar unit is located:

a. At the dispersal pad

b. At the tip of the bovie pencil

c. In the generator

d. In the insulated wire

b. At the tip of bovie pencil

The stapling unit that produces a double staggered row of staples and cuts through tissue is a(n):

a. TA

b. EEA

c. GIA

d. ligating clip

c. GIA

The type of suture that loses tensile strength in 5 to 10 days is:

a. Vicryl

b. Surgical gut

c. Chromic gut

d. Surgical Silk

a. Surgical gut

The position with the patient supine and the head tilted down is:

a. Trendelenburg

b. Reverse Trendelenburg

c. Modified fowlers

d. Kraske

a. Trendelenburg

For a cesarean section, the patient is positioned:

a. supine, with the feet slightly elevated

b. lithotomy

c. supine with the right side slightly elevated

d. supine with the left side slightly elevated

c. Supine with the right side slightly elevated

An example of res ipsa loquitor would be:

a. Unsigned consent

b. Patient record given to an unauthorized person

c. Leaving the patient alone in a hallway

d. Leaving a raytec in the patient

d. Leaving a raytec in the patient

The pathway around the nucleus that the electrons follow is called the:

a. valence shell

b. conduit

c. Atomic current

d. frequency cycle

a. valence shell

An expression of the relationship that one property has to another is:

a. proportion

b. ratio

c. percentage

d. fraction

b. ratio

During a sentinel node biopsy, the surgeon will inject:

a. hypaque

b. methylene blue

c. lymphazurin

d. isovue

c. lymphazurin

Which structure(s) are removed during a tonsillectomy:

a. Palatine tonsils

b. adenoid tonsils

c. pharyngeal tonsils

d. laryngeal and pharyngeal tonsils

a. Palatine tonsils

A burn that involves epidermis and part of the dermis is classified as:

a. first degree

b. second degree

c. third degree

d. fourth degree

b. second degree

The proximal and distal ends of a long bone are:

a. diaphysis

b. metaphysic

c. epiphysis

d. condyle

c. epiphysis

The type of saw used for limb amputation is a(n):

a. oscillating saw

b. reciprocating saw

c. skeeter saw

d. dubousset saw

a. oscillating saw

A keller procedure is used to correct:

a. hammer toe

b. hallux valgus

c. bakers cyst

d. colles fracture

b. hallux valgus

Nearsightedness is:

a. hyperopia

b. astigmatism

c. myopia

d. microtia

c. myopia

When preparing ratcheted instruments for sterilization, what should the surgical technologist do:

a. close ratchets

b. soak instrument in normal saline for 10 minutes prior to assembling

c. place grossly contaminated instruments into the ultrasonic cleaner

d. leave ratchets open

d. leave ratchets open

Which connective tissue connects bone to bone:

a. tendon

b. ligament

c. fascia

d. cartilage

b. ligament

Volvulus is a condition describing:

a. prolapse of the uterus

b. telescoping of the intestine

c. twisting of the bowel

d. herniation of the bowel

c. twisting of the bowel

An agent used to identified diseased tissue in the cervix is:

a. Lugols solution

b. methylene blue

c. tannic acid
d. conization

a. Lugols solution

The surgical removal of a fluid filled sac in the tunica vaginalis is:
a. Bartholin's cyst excision
b. hydrocelectomy
c. varicocelectomy
d. hydrocystectomy

b. hydrocelectomy

A patient suffering from prognathism has a(n):
a. receding chin
b. imbalance between the sides of the face
c. projecting jaw
d. open bite

c. projecting jaw

Microtia can be corrected with which surgical procedure?
a. Mentoplasty
b. Palatoplasty
C. Cheiloplasty
d. Otoplasty

d. Otoplasty

The spleen is located in the
a. right hypochondriac region
b. right epigastric region

c. left hypochondriac region
d. left epigastric region

c. left hypochondriac region

The medical term denoting rupture is
a. -rrhexis
b. -pexy
c. -rrhagia
d. –rrhaphy

a. -rrhexis

The gland that is both endocrine and exocrine is the
a. spleen
b. liver
c. pituitary
d. pancreas

d. pancreas

The medication used to treat malignant hyperthermia is
a. Diprovan
b. Protamine
c. Dantrolene
d. Lidocaine

c. Dantrolene

The second phase of wound healing is
a. Lag phase
b. Maturation

c. Proliferation
d. Granulation

c. Proliferation

Polygalactin 910 is
a. Monocryl
b. Vicryl
c. Maxon
d. PDS II

b. Vicryl

The instrument that uses ultrasonic energy to cut and coagulate simultaneously is the
a. CUSA
b. LASER
c. Harmonic Scalpel
d. Cyrotherapy Unit

c. Harmonic Scalpel

A Billroth II is a(n)
a. Gastrojejunostomy
b. Gastroduodenostomy
c. Total gastrectomy
d. Biliopancreatic diversion

a. Gastrojejunostomy

Endoscopic visualization of the peritoneal cavity is a(n)
a. colonoscopy
b. laparoscopy

c. arthroscopy

d. cystoscopy

b. laparoscopy

A rotator cuff tear occurs in the

a. knee

b. elbow

c. shoulder

d. ankle

c. shoulder

Bacteria that lives and grows best in decreased is classified as

a. aerobic

b. anaerobic

c. bacilli

d. clostridium

b. anaerobic

Putti-Platt is procedure to correct

a. rotator cuff repair

b. AC joint separation

c. Humeral fracture

d. Recurrent anterior shoulder dislocation

d. recurrent anterior shoulder dislocation

The Galea is located in the

a. Abdomen

b. Scalp

c. Upper leg
d. Back

b. scalp

The eight Cranial nerve is the
a. Vagus
b. Vestibulocochlear
c. Trigeminal
d. Abducens

b. Vestibulocochlear

Continuous sutures is also referred to as a(n)
a. Running stitch
b. Purse string
c. Retention suture
d. Buried suture

a. Running stitch

A mayo needle
a. is swaged
b. is less traumatic
c. is closed eyed
d. is a control release

c. is closed eyed

During an inguiinal hernia repair, the vas deferens is retracted with a(n)
a. Army-Navy
b. Red Robinson Catheter

c. Silastic tubing
d. Penrose drain

d. Penrose drain

The most common site for hernia formation is at this anatomical site
a. Hesselbach's triangle
b. Umbilicus
c. Poupart's ligmanet
d. Diaphragm

a. Hesselbach's triangle

Pneumoperitoneum is created with this gas
a. Carbon monoxide
b. Nitrous
c. Carbon dioxide
d. Oxygen

a. Carbon dioxide

A simple Mastectomy involves:
a. Removal of the entire breast and associated lymph nodes
b. Removal of the breast without lymph node dissection
c. Removal of breast and axillary contents
d. Removal of only affected breast tissue with preservation of the remaining tissue

b. Removal of the breast without lymph node dissection

The position for a patient undergoing excision of Zenker's diverticulum will be
a. Supine
b. Prone

c. Lateral

d. Semi-fowlers

d. Semit-flowers

The hormone that is present in as few as 10 days after conception is

a. Human Chorionic Gonadotropin

b. Luteinizing Hormone

c. Progesterone

d. Prolactin

a. Human Chorionic Gonadotropin

Protamine Sulfate reverses the effects of

A. Epinephrine

b. Narcotics

c. Metabolic acidosis

d. Heparin

d. Heprine

A Jackson Pratt is a(n)

a. Sump drain

b. Closed vacuum drain

c. Gravity drain

d. Cigarette drain

b. Closed vacuum drain

What is the most likely LASER to be used in conjunction with a Cystoscope?

a. Holmium:YAG

b. Xenon

c. Krypton

d. YAG

a. Holmium: YAG

Atelectasis is

a. Inflammation of mucous membranes

b. Stasis of peristalsis post operatively

c. Collapsed lung

d. Dehiscence of a wound

c. Collapsed lung

A common post operative complaint after laparoscopic procedures is

a. Size of incision

b. Chest pain

c. Back pain

d. Shoulder pain

d. Shoulder pain

The patient position for a perineal prostatectomy is

a. Supine

b. Lithotomy

c. Exaggerated lithotomy

d. Kraske

c. Exaggerated lithotomy

The creation of a nasoantral window in the maxillary bone to remove diseased tissue and drain sinuses is a(n)

a. Caldwell Luc

b. Submucosa Resection

c. FESS

d. UPPP

a. Caldwell Luc

An example of a nonadherent dressing is

a. Adaptic

b. Cloth tape

c. Tegaderm

d. Steri-strips

a. Adaptic

Club foot is a condition known as

a. Coxa vera

b. Talipes equinovarus

c. Exostosis

d. Dupuytrens Contracture

b. Talipes equinovarus

A hip case from waist to toes on the affected side and from the waist to knee on the unaffected side is a(n)

a. Cylinder cast

b. Long limb cast

c. Body cast

d. Spica cast

d. Spica cast

A double bowl shaped glass evacuator used in bladder surgery is a(n)

a. Toomey
b. Ellik
c. Closed vacuum drain
d. Iglesias

b. Ellik

Hair-like extensions responsible for movement of fluid around cells are

a. Flagella
b. Pili
C. Cilia
d. Pseudopods

c. Cilia

The only bone in the body that does not articulate with another bone is the

a. Patella
b. Mandible
c. Incus
d. Hyoid

d. Hyoid

The valve separating the right atrium and the right ventricle is the

a. Tricuspid
b. Mitral
c. Pulmonary
d. Semi-lunar

a. Tricuspid

The first phase of general anesthesia is
a. recovery
b. maintenance
c. induction
d. emergence

c. induction

All of the following are factors influencing chemical disinfection EXCEPT
a. Exposure time
b. Pounds of steam pressure (psi)
c. Amount of Bioburden present
d. pH

B. Pounds of steam pressure (psi)

A positioning device for modified prone position is a(n)
a. Wilson frame
b. bean bags
c. adhesive tape
d. kidney rest

a. Wilson frame

Which of the following is a non-absorbable synthetic monofilament suture:
a. polygalactin 910
b. monocryl
c. prolene
d. PDS

c. Prolene

The instrument not commonly found on a D&C set is:

a. Randall stone forceps

b. Dilators

c. sound

d. Weitlaner

d. Weitlaner

The congenital defect where the vertebrae do not close leaving the spinal cord unprotected is:

a. myleomengocele

b. spina bifida

c. arteriovenous malformation

d. Menier's disease

b. spina bifida

Which instrument is a urethral sound?

a. Hegar

b. Sims

c. Van buren

d. Mason Judd

C. Van buren

Whipple procedure is done to treat:

a. pancreatic cancer

b. obesity

c. stomach cancer

d. enlarged spleen

a. pancreatic cancer

Which structure is not ligated and divided during a cholecystectomy?

a. cystic duct

b. cystic artery

c. hepatic duct

d. cystic vein

C. hepatic duct

Anectine is a(n):

a. non-depolarizing muscle relaxant

b. depolarizing muscle relaxant

c. neuroleptanalgesic

d. sedative

b. depolarizing muscle relaxant

Bakers cyst are found:

a. in the stomach

b. behind the patella

c. in the elbow

d. in the popliteal fossa

d. in the popliteal fossa

The most common incision for cesarean section is:

a. Pfannenstiel

b. transverse

c. midline

d. Mcburneys

a. Pfannenstiel

A component of effective communication is:

a. speaking for others

b. defending a stance

c. using open ended sentences

d. working independently

c. using open ended sentences

The common approach for a simple mastoidectomy is:

a. Transnasal

b. anterior neck

c. postaural

d. transmaxillae

c. postaural

The sequence for screw placement is:

a. drill, tap, measure, insert screw

b. measure, drill, tap, insert screw

c. drill, insert screw

d. drill, measure, tap, insert screw

d. drill, measure, tap, insert screw

Cadaver bone is considered:

A. autograft

b. homograft

c. allograft

d. heterograft

b. homograft

PDS is a(n):
a. absorbable, synthetic monofilament suture
b. nonabsorbable, synthetic monofilament suture
c. absorbable, synthetic multifilament suture
d. nonabsorbable, synthetic multifilament suture

a. absorbable, synthetic monofilament suture

Cheyne-stokes respiration is:
a, wheezing sounds due to an obstruction
b. deep, gasping respiration indicative of a diabetic coma
c. irregular breathing due to apnea or hyperpena
d. rattling or bubbling sounds when breathing

c. irregular breathing due to apnea or hyperpena

Which surgical procedure would be performed with the patient in the lateral position?
a. pilonidal cystectomy
b. lumbar laminectomy
c. hiatal hernia repair
d. total hip arthroplasty

d. total hip arthroplasty

A contaminated case with an infection rate of 15% to 20% wound be classified as:
a. class 1
b. class 2
c. class 3
d. class 4

C. class 3

Which side of a sterile wrapper is opened first?

a. the far side

b. the left side

c. the right side

d. the near side

a. the far side

The instrument that measures intraocular pressure is a(n):

a. wicker caliper

b. Schiotz tonometer

c. taylor sphygmomanometer

d. Wescott keratometer

b. Schiotz tonometer

The condition where there is a separation of the retina from the choroid is:

a. retinopathy

b. retinal detachment

c. retinol deficiency

d. retinal layer idiopathic syndrome

b. retinal detachment

The innermost layer of the uterus is the:

a. myometrium

b. perimetrium

c. endometrium

d. mucous membrane

c. endometrium

An example of a hinge joint is the:

a. elbow

b. hip

c. wrist

d. thumb

a. elbow

The body's first line of defense against microbial infect is :

a. white blood cells

b. lymph

c. antigen/antibody reaction

d. unbroken skin

d. unbroken skin

To reduce the risk of fire when using LASERs, what precaution should be used?

a. use an alcohol prep that dries quickly

b. use an open oxygen system

c. moisten sponges around target tissue

d. have a class A extinguisher available

c. moisten sponges around target tissue

A solid state has:

a. A fixed volume

b. will expand to fit space

c. has a solvent

d. has no fixed shape

a. a fixed volume

A single robotic arm is used to:

a. translate surgeons hand movements

b. perform remote surgery

c. manipulate endoscopic telescopes

d. control room functions

c. manipulate endoscopic telescopes

How are permanent specimens sent to pathology?

a. dry

b. in 10% formalin

c. without solution

d. on a sponge

b. in 10% formalin

The thoracic lymphatic duct drains into:

a. the right jugular vein

b. the left jugular vein

c. the right subclavian vein

d. the left subclavian vein

d. the left subclavian vein

An agent given to combat metabolic acidosis is:

a. Sodium bicarbonate

b. magnesium sulfate

c. potassium chloride

d. albumin

a. Sodium bicarbonate

A patient in the prone position without proper padding is at risk for:

a. lower leg emboli

b. hyperextension of the head

c. pressure on the vena cava and abdominal aorta

d. compartment syndrome

c. pressure on the vena cava and abdominal aorta

Steam sterilizers are tested with the spore forming bacteria called:

a. bacillus subtilis

b. bacillus stearothermophilus

c. bacillus palladium

d. bacillus shingellosis

b. bacillus stearothermophilus

Which of the following is true about prepping?

a. prep "dirty" areas first

b. prep "clean" areas first

c. use one prep kit for two clean areas

d. do not use prep solutions of the face

b. prep "clean" areas first

in robotics, Roll refers to:

a. movement to the right

b. movement to the left

c. rotation

d. movement upward

c. rotation

Which statement is true about microinstrumentation?

a. they have a dull finish

b. they are straight

c. they cannot be flashed

d. they cannot be placed in the ultrasonic cleaner

a. they have a dull finish

Hepatitis B is a:

a. staphylococcal bacterium

b. streptococcal bacterium

c. vibrios

d. virus

d. virus

the masseter muscle is used when:

a. flexing the head

b. abducting the arm

c. chewing

d. closing the eyes

c. chewing

which of the following is a thoracic retractor?

a. davidson

b. greenburg

c. sauerbruch

d. sarot

a. davidson

the medication administered after eye surgery to rapidly constrict the pupil is:

a. miostat

b. miochol

c. mydriacyl

d. Diamox

b. miochol

The Leyla-yasergil retractor is used in which specialty surgery:

a. orthopedics

b. ophthalmic

c. pediatrics

d. neurosurgery

d. neurosurgery

Which of the following is a bone holding forcep?

a. chandler

b. lowman

c. murphy

d. hibbs

b. lowman

A possible complication of radical prostatectomy is:

a. impotence

b. testicular torsion

c. uremia

d. kidney stones

a. impotence

Wilms' tumors occur in the:

a. abdomen

b. popliteal fossa

c. kidneys

d. testes

c. kidneys

Intussusceptions may require:

a. gastrectomy

b. hemicolectomy

c. small bowel resection

d. pyloroplasty

c. small bowel resection

the incision that is made between two rectus abdominis muscles, continues down the linea alba and curves around the umbilicus is a:

a. transverse

b. midline

c. paramedian

d. kocher

b. midline

Wertheim procedure with abdominoperineal resection is called:

a. anterior exenteration

b. radical hysterectomy

c. posterior exenteration

d. vesicourethral exenteration

C. posterior exenteration

According to Erickson's developmental stages, trust versus mistrust occurs at:
a. 0-1 year
b. 12-18 years
c. 18-30 years
d. 2-5 years

a. 0-1 years

An institutional accreditation for allied health programs is:
a. JCAHO
b. AMA
c. ANSI
d. CAAHEP

D. CAAHEP

the causative agent of thrush is:
a. mold
b. yeast
c. bacteria
d. parasites

b. yeast

injusry sustained by the patient due to activity of health care providers is called:
a. iatrogenic injury
b. assault
c. negligence
d. contributory injury

b. assault

Surgical patients recover in:
a. The ICU
b. Pre-op holding areas
c. PACU
d. critical care unit

c. PACU

Surgical stainless teel would most likely be used for:
a. abdominal closures
b. cardiovascular procedures
c. general closures
d. Sternal closures

d. Sternal closures

The most likely needle for use in the liver would be:
a. cutting
b. blunt
c. taper
d. reverse cutting

b. blunt

Water for plaster cast application should be:
a. warm
b. cool
c. room temperature
d. hot

c. room temperature

the suture line used to close the appendix stump is:

a. purse-string

b. continuous

c. interrupted

d. mattress

a. purse-string

a FESS is:

a. abdominal surgery

b. orthopedic surgery

c. sinus surgery

d. oral surgery

c. Sinus surgery

Rhotons are used in:

a. Vascular surgery

b. Neurosurgery

c. Ophthalmic surgery

c. Plastic surgery

b. Neurosurgery

The middle layer of the meninges is:

a. Pia

B. Dura

c. Neurilemma

d. Arachnoid

d. Arachnoid

-malcia is the medical term for:

a. softening

b. condition

c. enlargement

d. break down, dissolve

a. softening

Removal of the parathyroid glands may cause:

a. muscle weakness

b. tetany

c. Graves disease

d. hyperthyroidism

b. tetany

The gland that helps develop the immune system is the:

a. pituitary

b. thyroid

c. pineal

d. thymus

d. thymus

Colles fractures occur:

a. in the femur

b. in the ankle

c. in the wrist

d. in the humerous

c. in the wrist

Which in-situ vein is used for femoral popliteal bypass?

a. radial

b. femoral vein

c. popliteal vein

d. saphenous vein

d. saphenous vein

Arteriotomies are extended with:

a. 11 blade

b. Potts smith scissors

c. Metzenbaum scissors

d. Steven tenotomy scissors

b. Potts smith scissors

A common site for cerebral aneurysms is:

a. Circle of wills

b. Temporal lobe

c. Frontal lobe

d. Occipital lobe

a. Circle of wills

An osteosarcoma is a(n):

a. Benign bone tumor

b. malignant tumor of cartilage

c. malignant tumor of perisoteum

d. malignant bone tumor

d. malignant bone tumor

Z-plasty may be performed to correct:
a. Dupuytren's contracture
b. Syndactyly
c. Rhytidectomy
d. Rhinoplasty

a. Dupuytren's contracture

A verruca is a(n):
a. mole
b. boil
c. wart
d. skin ulcer

c. wart

Which anesthetic agent may be used in ENT surgeries:
a. Levophed
b. Dantrium
c. Fentanyl
d. Cocaine

d. Cocaine

Scar tissue caused by fibrous collagen is:
a. Cicatrix
b. Granulation
c. Keloid
d. Granuloma

b. Granulation

Sterilization by ethylene oxide takes:

a. 2-3 hours

b. 24 hours

c. 30 minutes

d. 4 minutes

a. 2-3 hours

A metal or plastic device that holds a carpule of medication is a(n):

a. toomey

b. tubex

c. leur loc

d. ampoule

b. tubex

Para- is the root word for:

a. behind

b. through

c. beside

d. beneath

c. Beside

A gunshot wound to the bowel would be closed with:

a. First intention wound healing

b. Granulation

c. Second intention wound healing

d. Third intention wound healing

d Third intention wound healing

Bowel technique involves:

a. Two set ups

b. Isolation of contaminated instruments

c. Passing contaminated instruments off the field

d. Creating a "safe zone" for contaminated instruments

b. Isolation of contaminated instruments

A patient undergoing an AAA would be placed in:

a. Supine position

b. Lateral position

c. Modified beachchair

d. Lithotomy position

a. Supine position

Arterial embolectomy will be cleared with a(n):

a. syringe

b. foley

c. t-tube

d. fogarty

d. fogarty

A Javid shunt may be used when performing:

a. CABG

b. Carotid endarterectomy

c. AV shunt

d. Peritonenjugular shunt

b. carotid endarterectomy

There are _____ extrinsic eye muscles:
a. 4
b. 5
c. 6
d. 7

c. 6

The temperature of a prevacuum sterilizer should be:
a. 250 degrees
b. 270 degrees
c. 200 degrees
d. 280 degrees

b. 270 degrees

Reglan is a(n):
a. Histamine blocker
b. Anesthetic
c. Antiemetic
d. Anticholinergic

c. Antiemetic

The series of fluid filled canals located in the temporal bone is the :
a. Vestibule
b. Cochlea
c. Osseous labyrinth
d. Semicircular canals

c. Osseous labryrinth

Elevated white blood cell count is referred to as:

a. Leukocytosis

b. Leukopenia

c. Leukoragia

d. Leukemia

a. Leukocytosis

An example of a narcotic antagonist agent is:

a. Lidocaine

b. Dantrolene

c. Narcan

d. Anectine

c. Narcan

The loss of heat due to collisions of molecules at different temperatures is called:

a. conduction

b. convection

c. radiation

d. gas diffusion

a. conduction

A footboard may be required of patients placed in the _____ position:

a. lithotmy

b. trendelenburg

c. kraske

d. reverse trendelenburg

d. reverse trendelenburg

The purpose of an indwelling urethral catheter for surgical procedures includes all of the following EXCEPT:

a. monitoring urine production
b. keep bladder irrigated
c. collect sterile specimens
d. keep bladder deflated

b. Keep bladder irrigated

Abnormal fibrous tissues that bind organs together are:

a. cohesions
b. epithelial granulation
c. adheasions
d. keloids

c. adhesions

Suture gauge refers to:

a. diameter of the suture strand
b. needle size
d. mulitfilament suture
d. tensile strength

a. diameter of the suture dtrand

X-ray visualization of the bladder using contrast media is a(n):

a. cystoscopy
b. cystogram
c. cystmetrogram
d. KUB

b. cystogram

Which of the following is an orthopedic instrument?

a. Fogarty clamp

b. Serrefines

c. Bennett

d. McPherson typing forcep

c. Bennett

Bleeding between the dura mater and the arachnoid is:

a. Epidural hematoma

b. Subdural hematoma

c. Subarachnoid hematoma

d. Intracerebral hematoma

b. Subdural hematoma

The association that develops medical device standards is:

a. AMA

b. ASPAN

c. NIOSH

d. AAMI

a. AAMI

The term that is used when an infant's head is to large to pass through the pelvis to the mother is:

a. Cephalopelvic disproportion

b. Cephalodystocia

c. Cephalophalic disproportion

d. Hyperemisis gravidarum

a. Cephalopelvic disproportion

Bougies and balloon dilators may be used to treat:
a. hypospadia
b. urethral stenosis
c. Vesicourethral reflux
d. Phimosis

b. Urethral stenosis

The highest level of Maslow's Hierarchy is:
a. Self-esteem
b. Love and belonging
c. Self-actualization
d. Social affiliations

c. Self-actualization

The instrument used to grasp the cervix during a D&C is:
a. Sims uterine sound
b. Tenaculum
c. Auvard
d. Bozeman

b. Tenaculum

A three lumen tube is for:
a. Irrigation, aspiration and urine
b. Aspiration, escape of air and suction
c. Aspiration, irrigation and escape of air
d. Irrigation, urine and escape of air

c. Aspiration, irrigation and escape of air

The second stage loop colostomy is performed how long after the first stage?

a. 24 hours

b. 48 hours

c. 72 hours

d. 1 week

b. 48 hours

What should be done before patient catheterization?

a. test balloon

b. surgical prep

c. secure catheter to patient with tape

d. place patient in lithotomy position

a. test balloon

Which state is true regarding lateral positioning?

a. patient is placed on operative side

b. lower leg is flexed

c. arms are tucked

d. a minimum of 3 people must be present

b. lower leg is flexed

Aeger Primo means:

a. First, do no harm

b. Negligence

c. The things speaks for itself

d. Patient first

d. Patient first

The reason a specific drug should not be used is a(n):

a. side effect

b. indication

c. contraindication

d. adverse effect

c. contraindication

The flow of electrons back and forth along a single pathway due to changes in polarity is:

a. AC current

b. DC current

c. Voltage

d. Conductivity

a. AC current

A common complication of Diabetes Mellitus is:

a. Obesity

b. Infection

c. Malnourishment

d. Decreased blood clotting time

b. infection

The psi for gravity air displacement sterilization is:

a. Between 20 and 25

b. 27

c. Between 12 and 15

d. Between 15 and 17

d. Between 15 and 17

The biologic test for EO sterilization involves:

a. Bacillus stearothermophilus

b. Bacillus tetani

c. Bacillus subtilis

d. Clostridium difficile

c. Bacillus subtilis

Distension during hysteroscopy is commonly attained by:

a. Dextran

b. Sterile water

c. Saline

D. Albumin

a. Dextran

The series of canals found in compact bone that allows blood vessels and nerves to enter is called the:

a. Bursa system

b. Sharpeys fibers

c. Haversian system

d. Elysain system

c. Haversian system

Gtt is the abbreviation for:

a. Epiglottis

b. Grain

C. Drop

D. Tongue

C. Drop

The stapler which places a double row of staggered staples and has a cutting blade is a(n):

a. Skin stapler

b. TA

c. GIA

d. ILA (EEA)

C. GIA

The common bile duct joins the pancreatic duct at this anatomical structure:

a. Sphincter of Oddi

b. Duct of Wirsung

c. Ampulla of Vader

d. Pancreatic fundus

b. Duct of Wirsung

Which of the following instruments would be used for kidney removal?

a. Bailey

b. Kerrison

C. Woodson

d. Davidson

a. Bailey

Bletharochalasis is defined as:

A. Loss of elasticity of the skin of the eyelids

b. Lazy eye

c. Cross eyes

d. Peri-orbital fracture

a. Loss of elasticity of the skin of the eyelids

Intracranial aneurysms may be approached in all of the following ways EXCEPT:
a. Frontal
b. Bifrontal
c. Frontotemporal
d. Transphenoidal

d. Transphenoidal

When performing a lumpectomy, what should be removed?
a. The entire mass
b. The mass and lymph nodes
c. The mass and non-affected tissue margins
d. A small amount of tissue for pathology

c. The mass and non-affected margins

Temporalis fascia taken for tympanic membrane graft should:
a. be placed on a drying block
b. remain moist
c. be cut by the ST to the surgeons specifications
d. taken 24 hours prior to the surgery

a. be placed on a drying block

A self-retaining intracranial retractor is a(n):
a. beckman
b. Leyla
c. Israel
d. Omni

b. Leyla

A case where there is a major break in aspetic technique has the designation of:
a. Class I
b. Class II
c. Class III
d. Class IV

d. Class III

A flat latex drain used to retract the spermatic cord during inguinal hernia repair is:
a. sump drain
b. penrose drain
c. red robinson
d. tenkhof drain

b. penrose drain

Movement in and around the sterile field should be:
a. out of normal traffic flows
b. kept to a minimum
c. done freely
d. constricted to the anesthesia personnel

b. kept to a minimum

During a laparosocpic procedure, who manipulates the tower settings?
a. the surgeon
b. the anesthesiologist
c. the circulator under direction from the surgeon
b. the scrub under direction of the surgeon

c. the circulator under direction from the surgeon

Helminths are:

a. Fungal infections

b. Rickettsial agents

c. Protozoan parasites

d. Parasitic worms

d. Parasitic worms

Muscle irritability may be caused by a buildup of:

a. Lactic acid

b. Carbon dioxide

c. Calcium ions

d. Acetylcholine

a. Lactic acid

How many carpals are in each wrist?

a. 5

b. 8

c. 10

d. 16

b. 8

Which of the following is a blood thinner?

a. Thrombin

b. Ephedrine

c. Aspirin

d. Purodigin

c. Aspirin

Which of the following is true about surgical masks?

a. They should be worn either on or off, not around the neck

b. Two masks should be worn in active TB cases

c. Masks should be worn in semi-restricted areas

d. Masks should be put on before the buffant

a. They should be worn either on or off, not around the neck

Which tendon will be used as graft when repairing the flexor tendon:

a. Achilles

b. Palmaris longus

c. Extensor pollicis

d. Extensor carpi

b. Palmaris longus

KTP lasers are produced when Nd:YAG light is passed through a(n):

a. Ruby particulate plasma filter

b. Garnet crystal

c. Argon particle filter

d. Potassium titanium phosphate crystal

d. Potassium titanium phosphate crystal

Which of the following is not true about materials for gowns and drapes?

a. Material should provide microbial barrier

b. Material should be laundered

c. Non-woven material should be laundered and sterilized after each procedure

d. Woven material should be repaired with heat patches

c. Non-woven material should be laundered and sterilized after each procedure

The device that is used to measure blood pressure or pulse using ultrasonic high-frequency sound eaves is a(n):

a. Doppler
b. Spirometer
c. Insufflators
d. ECHO

A. Doppler

Glutaraldehyde requires an exposure time of _____ to achieve sterilization:

a. 20 minutes
b. 10 hours
c. 10 minutes
d. 5 hours

b. 10 hours

The suture most likely used on slow healing wounds where there is a need for wound support is:

a. Polyglactin 910
b. Chromic Gut
c. Polypropylene
d. Polydioxanone

d. Polydioxanone

A total Abdominal Hysterectomy wound remove which anatomical structure(s)?

a. Uterus, fallopian tubes and ovaries
b. Uterus and ovaries
c. Uterus
d. Uterus, fallopian tubes, ovaries, and upper third of the vaginal vault

c. Uterus

If a surgical blade is broken during a procedure, how should the Surgical Technologist handle the count?

a. The ST should discard the sharp in the sharps container

b. The count should reflect all parts of the broken blade

c. The count should remain the same, with the pieces counted as one

d. The circulating nurse will remove the blade from the room

b. The count should reflect all parts of the broken blade

Which of the following instruments would likely be found in a general set?

a. Gerald forceps

b. Bethune

c. Duvall

d. Curved Kocher

d. Curved Kocher

A portocaval shunt creates an anastomosis between the inferior vena cava and this structure:

a. Portal vein

b. Splenic vein

c. Superior mesenteric vein

d. Renal vein

a. Portal vein

Which of the following procedures is likely to require a drain post operatively?

a. Hysterectomy

b. Marsupialization of Bartholin's cyst

b. D&C

d. Inguinal hernia repair

b. Marsupialization of Barthonlin's cyst

The valve that separates the small intestine from the large intestine is the:

a. Pyloric valve

b. Ileocecal valve

c. Cardiac valve

d. Ampulla of Vater

b. Ileocecal valve

Cowpers Glands are associated with which anatomical structure:

a. Kidneys

b. Uterus

c. Bladder

d. Prostate

d. Prostate

Gore-tex grafts are made of:

a. Knitted polyester

b. Knitted velour

c. Polytetrafluoroethylene

d. Knitted polyester

c. Polytetrafluoroethylene

Packages of surgical instruments should not weigh more than:

a. 15 lb

b. 16 lb.

c. 18 lb.

d. 20 lb.

b. 16 lb

An example of a surgically clean, but not sterile, endoscopic procedure is:

a. Laparoscopic cholecystectomy

b. Thoracoscopy

c. Cystoscopy

d. Mediansinosocpy

c. Cystoscopy

A liver biopsy would most likely be done with a:

a. Toomey syringe

b. Jamshidi needle

c. Silverman

d. Tubex syringe

c. Silverman

Premature closure of cranial sutures is a condition called:

a. AV malformation

b. Hydrocephalus

c. Spina bifida

d. Craniosynostosis

d. Craniosynostosis

When anastomosing the renal vein during living donor procedures, which suture would most likely be used?

a. 5-0 double-armed vascular suture

b. 7-0 double-armed vicryl

c. 3-0 chromic

d. 6-0 single-armed bylon

a. 5-0 double-armed vascular suture

In the event of an incorrect count, which action should be taken immediately?
a. X-rays should be taken to locate the item
b. Anesthesia should be informed as the procedure will be delayed
c. Documentation must be completed
d. Inform the surgeon

d. Inform the surgeon

The generic form of Marcaine is:
a. Xylocaine
b. Bupivicaine
c. Mepivicaine
d. Tetracaine

b. Bupivicaine

The toxins that are produced by bacteria and are released upon destruction of the cells are considered:
a. Exotoxins
b. Myotoxins
c. Endotoxins
d. Fibrinolysins

c. Endotoxins

The fold of peritoneum that hangs like an apron over the abdominal organs is called:
a. Mesentery
b. Omentum
c. Visceral peritoneal folds
d. Patietal peritoneal folds

b. Omentum

A benign cyst of the ovary containing contents from old blood is called a(n):
a. Carcinoma in situ
b. Dermoid cyst
c. Cystocele
d. Chocolate cyst

d. Chocolate cyst

An example of a motor driven dermatome is a(n):
a. Padgett
b. Hudson brace
c. Reese
d. Padgett-hood

a. Padgett

Burns are classified as electrical, thermal, chemical, and:
a. Dermal
b. Mechanical
c. Solid
d. Accelerant

b. Mechanical

When transporting a patient on a stretcher, you should:
a. push from the feet
b. push from the sides
c. push from the head
d. pull from the head

c. push from the head

Which of the following is a cephalosporin:

a. Garamycin

b. doxycycline

c. Omnipen

d. Ancef

d. Ancef

Which of the following is not true about activated glutaraldehyde?

a. Items must be damp when placed in solution

b. It must be monitored for concentration

c. It must be stored in a closed container

d. Gloves and goggles must be worn when working with Glutaraldehyde

a. Items must be damp when placed in solution

A non-invasive method to measure anesthesia levels is:

a. Urinary output

b. Blood pressure

c. Bispectral index

d. Pulmonary artery pressure

c. Bispectral index

A seamless tubular cotton dressing/drape is a(n):

a. Tubes

b. Ace

c. Coban

d. Stockinette

d. Stockinette

The three parts of a needle are point, body, and:

a. diameter

b. eye

c. size

d. code

b. eye

A common intestinal suture is:

a. 3-0 silk

b. 4-0 vicryl

c. 6-0 double armed prolene

d. 2 PDS II

a. 3-0 sile

During a Nissen Fundoplication, the fundus of the stomach is anchored against which anatomical structure:

a. 8th rib

b. Xyphoid process

c. Diaphragm

d. Esophagus

c. Diaphragm

A contraindication for hysterosocpy is:

a. lost IUD

b. Pregnancy

c. Infertility

d. Abnormal uterine bleeding

b. Pregnancy

Which surgical procedure may be done while sitting?

a. carpal tunnel release

b. craniotomy

c. SMR

d. excision of pressure sores

a. carpal tunnel release

A daily test used to check the veracity of Prevacuum sterilizers is:

a. Spore strip

b. Chemical indicator

c. Bowie dick

d. Schillers test

c. Bowie dick

A common suture for subcuticular closure is:

a. Monocryl

b. Nylon

c. Mersilene

d. Polydek

a. Monocryl

Factors that determine whether an individual will contract a disease post-exposure include all of the following EXCEPT:

a. Virulence

b. Duration of exposure

c. Resistance of host

d. Weight of host

d. Weight of host

The space between the cochlea and the semicircular canals of the inner ear is the:

a. Labyrinth

b. Anterior cavity

c. Vestibule

d. Auricle

C. Vestibule

A pressure point for someone placed in the prone position is the:

a. Sacrum

b. Lesser trochanter

c. Scapula

d. Lateral Knee

d. Lateral knee

The curette commonly used for endocervical scrapping is a(n):

a. Kervorkian

b. Thomas

c. Bozeman

d. Loop

a. Kervorkian

The stage of osteogenesis that creates a fibrous tissue and cartilage mesh is the:

a. Remodeling stage

b. Osteoid stage

c. Hematoma formation

d. Callus stage

d. Callus stage

Demerol is an example of a(n):
a. Inhalation anesthetic
b. Narcotic sedative
c. Antianxiety medication
d. Neuromusclar blocker

b. Narcotic sedative

failure of an organ to develop properly is called:
a. Atresia
b. Hypoplasia
c. Aplasia
d. Anaplasia

c. Aplasia

The chemical produced by a cell infected with viral particles that protects other cells is:
a. Interferon
b. Interlukin
c. Antitoxin
d. Antiserum

a. Interferon

Relative humidity in the OR should be maintained at:
a. 55-60%
b. 50-55%
c. 60-65%
d. 45-50%

b. 50-55%

The suture line for inner layers of bowel mucosa is:
a. Pursestring
b. Limbert
c. Halstead
d. Connel

d. Connel

The gas used to inflate the peritoneum during laparoscopic procedures is:
a. Carbon dioxide
b. Oxygen
c. Carbon monoxide
d. Nitrous oxide

a. Carbon dioxide

A common drain used for cholecystostomy is:
a. Fogarty
b. Pezzar
c. Foley
d. Penrose

b. Pezzar

In the event of an incorrect count, which action should be taken immediately?
a. X-rays should be taken to locate the item
b. Anesthesia should be informed as the procedure will be delayted
c. Documentation must be completed
d. Inform the surgeon

d. Inform the surgeon

Sterile supplies and instruments for a case have been opened in OR 1. A surgical technologist was just informed that the case has been moved to OR 2 and the next case in OR 1 is scheduled in two hours. Which of the following is the BEST course of action?

A. Cover the sterile field with a sterile drape and move it from OR 1 to OR 2.
B. New sterile supplies and instruments should be obtained for OR 2 and the setup in OR 1 should be disposed of.
C. OR 1 should be left so that these supplies and instruments can be used by the next case.
D. The surgical technologist should argue that the procedure be held in OR 1 as planned.

B. New sterile supplies and instruments should be obtained for OR 2 and the setup in OR 1 should be disposed of.

Which of the following is the body's local tissue reaction to injury?
A. fever
B. infection
C. inflammation
D. immune reaction

C. inflammation

Which of the following instruments is used for a common bile duct exploration?
A. Fogarty clamp
B. Randall forceps
C. Pennington clamp
D. Forester ring forceps

B. Randall forceps

Which of the following is the MOST important consideration when cutting suture?

A. avoiding the knot
B. using sharp scissors

C. opening the scissors wide when cutting

D. tagging the end of suture to be cut with a hemostat

A. avoiding the knot

Which of the following structures are ligated and divided during the cholecystectomy?

A. cystic artery and cystic duct

B. hepatic artery and hepatic duct

C. cystic artery and common bile duct

D. hepatic artery and pancreatic duct

A. cystic artery and cystic duct

Which of the following may be used when applying a sterile dressing to a skin graft site?

A. pressure dressing

B. ABD pad

C. 4x4s

D. Steri-Strips

A. pressure dressing

When performing a dilation and curettage, which of the following instruments is used to grasp the cervix?

A. Sims

B. Auvard

C. Schroeder

D. Bozeman

C. Schroeder

On the way into the operating room, a terminally ill patient tells the nurse, "No matter what happens, it will be okay." Which of the Five Stages of Grief is the patient MOST likely in?

A. denial
B. bargaining
C. depression
D. acceptance

D. acceptance

Which of the following instruments is used for placement of cottonoid strips during a craniotomy?

A. bayonet forceps
B. Russian forceps
C. Kelly clamp
D. angled DeBakey clamp

A. bayonet forceps

When two individuals in sterile attire pass one another in the sterile field, they should
A. pass back-to-back.
B. both face the wall.
C. pass side-to-side.
D. both face the sterile field.

A. pass back-to-back.

Which of the following is used to oxygenate and circulate blood?
A. Doppler ultrasound
B. defibrillator
C. extracorporeal bypass
D. autotransfuser

C. extracorporeal bypass

The PRIMARY consideration in selecting an appropriate anesthetic agent is the
A. physiologic condition of the patient.
B. length of the procedure.
C. type of the procedure.
D. anxiety level of the patient.

A. physiologic condition of the patient.

If two basins are wrapped together for sterilizing, they should be packaged with one basin
A. stacked inside the other and separated by impervious material.
B. on its side and the other upside down.
C. stacked inside the other and wrapped in a towel.
D. stacked inside the other and separated by a towel.

D. stacked inside the other and separated by a towel.

Which of the following items may be used in positioning a patient for a total hip arthroplasty?
A. fracture table
B. Wilson frame
C. Andrews frame
D. bean bag

D. bean bag

A surgical technologist sees a neighbor being admitted. How should the surgical technologist respond?
A. Acknowledge the neighbor.
B. Reassure the neighbor that everything will be fine.
C. Do not acknowledge the neighbor unless greeted first.
D. Ignore the neighbor, even if greeted.

C. Do not acknowledge the neighbor unless greeted first

Instruments that come in contact with the appendiceal stump during an appendectomy should be

A. placed in a separate basin.
B. wiped with a saline sponge.
C. returned to the Mayo stand.
D. wiped with an alcohol sponge.

A. placed in a separate basin.

Which of the following is the MOST serious complication of a strangulated hernia?
A. shock
B. necrosis
C. infection
D. hemorrhage

B. necrosis

Which of the following techniques is NOT acceptable for draping the patient?
A. Hold the drapes high until directly over the patient.
B. Protect the gloved hands by cuffing the drapes.
C. Readjust the drapes as necessary after placement.
D. Place the drapes on a dry area.

C. Readjust the drapes as necessary after placement.

Which of the following structures is separated first when a paramedian incision is performed?
A. peritoneum
B. transverse abdominis

C. external oblique
D. rectus abdominis

D. rectus abdominis

Which of the following is MOST likely to be used to stabilize a cervical fracture?
A. Kirschner wire
B. Hoffman device
C. Steinmann pins
D. Mayfield clamp

D. Mayfield clamp

During a transurethral resection of the prostate, bleeding is controlled by
A. Gelfoam.
B. irrigation.
C. cauterization.
D. suture ligature.

C. cauterization.

To prevent contamination at the end of a surgical procedure, which of the following should be removed LAST by the surgical technologist in the scrub role?
A. patient's drapes
B. surgical gloves
C. surgical gown
D. Mayo stand drape

B. surgical gloves

In order to remove a portion of the kidney, the surgeon must enter which of the following?

A. synovial membrane

B. Gerota's fascia

C. Hesselbach's triangle

D. suprapleural membrane

B. Gerota's fascia

Which of the following is the MOST common straight catheter used prior to laparoscopic gynecological surgery in the OR?

A. Foley

B. Pezzer

C. Malecot

D. Robinson

D. Robinson

A Stamey needle is used for which of the following types of surgery?

A. hysterectomy

B. prostatectomy

C. bladder suspension

D. anterior colporrhaphy

C. bladder suspension

Immediately before a hemorrhoidectomy, which of the following procedures might be performed on the patient in the operating room?

A. cystoscopy

B. culdoscopy

C. sigmoidoscopy

D. laparoscopy

C. sigmoidoscopy

Which of the following is a fenestrated drape?

A. a drape with an opening that allows exposure of the operative site
B. a split drape that has two tails
C. a drape used to cover the operating table, instrument table, and body regions
D. an incise drape that is self-adhering

A. a drape with an opening that allows exposure of the operative site

An appendectomy incision closed using suture is considered to be which of the following types of wound closure?

A. primary intention
B. secondary intention
C. tertiary intention
D. third intention

A. primary intention

Which of the following patients is MOST likely to acquire a nosocomial infection?
A. a healthy female patient who is 45 years of age

B. a female patient in labor and delivery
C. a healthy male patient who is 45 years of age
D. a male patient who has diabetes

D. a male patient who has diabetes

31
The appendiceal stump, when inverted, is held in place by which of the following types of

suture?

A. mattress
B. traction
C. interrupted
D. purse-string

D. purse-string

Aerobic organisms are BEST characterized as

A. pathogenic.
B. nonpathogenic.
C. oxygen-requiring.
D. non-oxygen-requiring.

C. oxygen-requiring.

The PRIMARY purpose of chest tubes is to

A. irrigate the pleural space.
B. eliminate chest leaks.
C. prevent pulmonary emboli.
D. re-establish negative pressure.

D. re-establish negative pressure.

Which of the following is a surgical instrument designed for retracting?

A. Potts
B. Penfield
C. Lowman
D. Gelpi

D. Gelpi

Which of the following surgical procedures may be used to remove a carcinoma from the head of the pancreas?

A. Heller
B. Whipple
C. Bankart
D. Billroth I

B. Whipple

A sterile item used with an electrosurgical unit is the

A. generator.
B. patient return electrode.
C. active electrode.
D. foot pedal.

C. active electrode

What is the desired effect of atropine sulfate when used as a preoperative medication?

A. drowsiness
B. pain relief
C. decreased anxiety
D. drying of secretions

D. drying of secretions

A postoperative total arthroplasty patient presents to the emergency department with severe throbbing pain, fever, and malaise. Which of the following is the likely diagnosis?

A. osteoarthritis
B. osteoporosis
C. osteomyelitis
D. osteomalacia

C. osteomyelitis

Which of the following is used to stabilize a fractured finger?
A. Rush rods
B. Hagie pins
C. Knowles pins
D. Kirschner wires

D. Kirschner wires

Which of the following is the primary purpose for changing into operating room attire?
A. to standardize uniforms
B. to prevent the of spread of microorganisms
C. to identify operating room personnel
D. to avoid damage to personal attire

B. to prevent the of spread of microorganisms

A surgical technologist is assigned to a room where the patient happens to be his neighbor. To protect patient confidentiality, the technologist should indicate that he knows the patient and
A. continue with the procedure.
B. request to be removed from the room.
C. discuss patient personal medical information.
D. inform the surgeon.

B. request to be removed from the room.

Mannitol (Osmitrol) is used in neurosurgical procedures to
A. prevent bleeding.
B. decrease intracranial pressure.
C. anesthetize the operative site.
D. fight possible postoperative infection.

B. decrease intracranial pressure.

Which of the following lies between the lung and the chest wall?

A. mediastinum

B. peritoneum

C. pleura

D. pericardium

C. pleura

Which of the following is applied as a nonadherent dressing?

A. adaptic

B. collodion

C. steri-strip

D. Elastoplast

A. adaptic

A Balfour is used in which of the following procedures?

A. tracheostomy

B. sigmoid resection

C. pulmonary decortication

D. stapedectomy

B. sigmoid resection

If the VII cranial nerve is severed, which of the following is the result?

A. loss of hearing

B. loss of vision

C. facial paralysis

D. impairment of eye muscles

C. facial paralysis

When assisting with the closure of a skin incision and operating the skin stapler, the surgical technologist in the scrub role is placing the staples through which two layers?

A. cuticular and subcuticular
B. subicular and subcutaneous
C. subcuticular and subcutaneous
D. subcutaneous and fascia

A. cuticular and subcuticular

During which of the following surgeries is a Meckel's diverticulum typically discovered?

A. esophagectomy
B. appendectomy
C. prostatectomy
D. varicocelectomy

B. appendectomy

Which of the following layers are transected when a subcostal flank incision is used for a nephrectomy?
A. pre-peritoneal fat
B. linea alba
C. oblique muscles
D. rectus abdominis muscle

C. oblique muscles

A perforator is used for which of the following procedures?
A. cordotomy

B. craniotomy

C. laminectomy

D. spinal fusion

B. craniotomy

In preparation for a cranial aneurysm, which of the following pieces of equipment would MOST likely be used?

A. microscope

B. cryoprobe

C. Jordan Day drill

D. Crutchfield tongs

A. microscope

During strabismus surgery, which of the following is the first tissue layer that must be incised?
A. iris
B. cornea
C. sclera
D. conjunctiva

D. conjunctiva

When can instrument counts be omitted?

A. if an emergency procedure must be performed
B. when the surgical technologist in the circulator role becomes too busy
C. if instruments are needed in another operating room
D. when the patient is receiving outpatient surgery

A. if an emergency procedure must be performed

In which of the following positions is a patient placed for a right nephrectomy?

A. left lateral
B. right lateral
C. left lateral kidney
D. right lateral kidney

C. left lateral kidney

Which of the following examples illustrates UNSAFE technique for disposing of contaminated sharps?

A. Used suture needles and scalpel blades are removed from the needle counter and individually placed in the biohazard sharps container.
B. Used suture needles and scalpel blades remain in the needle counter and the closed needle counter is placed in the biohazard sharps container.
C. The biohazard sharps container is located as close as possible to the area in which the items were used.
D. Disposable surgical blades are removed from knife handles with a needle holder or other instrument.

A. Used suture needles and scalpel blades are removed from the needle counter and individually placed in the biohazard sharps container.

Why is the right kidney typically several centimeters lower than the left kidney?
A. The liver rests superior and anterior to the right kidney.
B. The liver rests superior and posterior to the right kidney.
C. The liver rests inferior and anterior to the right kidney.
D. The liver rests inferior and posterior to the right kidney.

A. The liver rests superior and anterior to the right kidney.

Which of the following should be the MINIMUM exposure time in a flash sterilizer for unwrapped instruments?

A. 1 minute
B. 3 minutes
C. 5 minutes
D. 7 minutes

B. 3 minutes

If a routine surgical procedure was performed without consent, the surgeon committed

A. assault.
B. battery.
C. malpractice.
D. liability.

B. battery.

If an adult patient refuses a blood transfusion, the surgical staff should

A. not administer blood to the patient.
B. administer blood only in an emergency.
C. administer blood only after sedation.
D. not perform any procedure that may require a transfusion.

A. not administer blood to the patient.

During the intraoperative phase, which of the following activities can be completed by both sterile and non-sterile members of the surgical team?

A. caring for the specimen
B. maintaining the patient's operative record

C. clearing residual blood from the surgical field
D. maintaining the sterile field and neutral zone

A. caring for the specimen

A lumbar meningocele involves removal of
A. cerebrospinal fluid.
B. lumbar disc.
C. meninges.
D. a fluid-filled sac.

D. a fluid-filled sac.

Wrinkle-free padding is applied to an extremity before application of a tourniquet to avoid

A. skin injuries.
B. improper inflation.
C. excessive blood loss.
D. skeletal injuries.

A. skin injuries

A specimen obtained for frozen section is generally removed from the sterile field intraoperatively because it
A. needs to be labeled by the circulator.
B. is sent to pathology immediately.
C. will contaminate the sterile field.
D. needs to be placed in formalin solution.

B. is sent to pathology immediately.

Which of the following procedures is used to visualize the cystic, hepatic, and common ducts?
A. barium enema

B. cholangiography

C. intravenous pyelography

D. upper gastrointestinal series

B. cholangiography

A scleral buckle procedure repairs

A. astigmatism.

B. detached retinas.

C. corneal scarring.

D. eye muscle contractures.

B. detached retinas.

Which of the following retractors should the surgical technologist have available to provide exposure to the patellar tendon while harvesting the graft for an ACL repair?

A. Senn
B. Richardson
C. Hayes
D. Fukuda

A. Senn

The surgical technologist in the scrub role should remain sterile following which of the following surgical procedures?
A. laparoscopic cholecystectomy
B. carotid endarterectomy
C. total hip arthroplasty
D. tympanoplasty

B. carotid endarterectomy

During dissection of the cystic duct in an open cholecystectomy, which of the following instruments is necessary?

A. Ochsner forceps

B. Jennings retractor

C. Mixter clamp

D. O'Sullivan-O'Connor retractor

C. Mixter clamp

A patient entering the operating room for a laparoscopic cholecystectomy looks jaundiced. Which of the following is the BEST explanation for this?

A. pancreatitis

B. biliary obstruction

C. cholecystitis

D. gastroschisis

B. biliary obstruction

The primary purpose of a local anesthetic is to

A. lower skin temperature.

B. reduce fear and anxiety.

C. block peripheral nerve receptors.

D. decrease bleeding.

C. block peripheral nerve receptors.

Which of the following is the correct skin preparation for a female patient undergoing a right mastectomy with possible axillary dissection?

A. shoulder, upper arm and extending down to the elbow, axilla, chest to the table line, and to the left shoulder

B. base of the neck, shoulder, scapula, chest to midline, and circumference of upper arm down to the elbow

C. entire arm, shoulder, axilla, including the hand

D. chin to umbilicus and laterally to the table line

A. shoulder, upper arm and extending down to the elbow, axilla, chest to the table line, and to the left shoulder

When performing a parotidectomy, which of the following nerves is identified and preserved with the use of a nerve stimulator?

A. facial nerve

B. recurrent laryngeal nerve

C. acoustic nerve

D. vagus nerve

A. facial nerve

Which of the following medications is the anesthesia provider responsible for recording the name, amount, and delivery method during a surgical procedure?

A. thrombin

B. topically applied epinephrine

C. polymyxin B sulfate irrigation

D. propofol

D. propofol

As a surgical technologist begins to prep a female patient for Foley catheterization, a bulge in the vaginal wall is noticed. Which of the following would cause this bulge?

A. cystocele

B. endometriosis

C. leiomyoma

D. ectopic pregnancy

A. cystocele

A surgical technologist enters the OR after scrubbing and notices spots of blood on the OR lights. Which of the following actions is the MOST appropriate?

A. Ignore the spots because they are small.

B. Tell the circulator to obtain replacements and wait at the scrub sink.

C. Ask the circulator to clean the spot and then proceed.

D. Break scrub to clean the lights and help open a new sterile field.

D. Break scrub to clean the lights and help open a new sterile field.

Which of the following instruments should be included in a transurethral resection of the prostate (TURP) setup?

A. lithotrite

B. urethrotome

C. resectoscope

D. Randall

C. resectoscope

Which of the following instruments has teeth?

A. Kocher

B. Mixter

C. Babcock

D. Mosquito

A. Kocher

☐☐

When entering the abdominal cavity, which of the following BEST describes the order of contact with the layers of tissue?
A. skin, fascia, subcutaneous, peritoneum, muscle
B. skin, subcutaneous, muscle, fascia, peritoneum
C. skin, fascia, peritoneum, subcutaneous, muscle
D. skin, subcutaneous, fascia, muscle, peritoneum

D. skin, subcutaneous, fascia, muscle, peritoneum

If a Kelly clamp is left in a patient who underwent a cholecystectomy, which of the following legal concepts apply?
A. misdemeanor
B. res ipsa loquitur
C. extension doctrine
D. intentional tort

B. res ipsa loquitur

A surgical technologist just opened an instrument set that is wet inside after undergoing steam sterilization. Which of the following is the MOST likely reason for the condensate in the package and how can it be corrected?
A. There are not enough instruments in the tray to allow for revaporization of the condensate. The number of instruments in the tray should be increased and the tray should be reprocessed.
B. The instrument set contained absorbant towels, which soaked up the moisture and prevented efficient drying. The tray should be reprocessed without any towels.
C. The absorbent towels were wrapped too tightly around the instrument tray, so they retained moisture. The tray should be reprocessed with loosely wrapped new towels.
D. Condensate has built up on the steam lines. The surgical technologist should clean the steam lines and reprocess the instrument tray.

C. The absorbent towels were wrapped too tightly around the instrument tray, so they retained moisture. The tray should be reprocessed with loosely wrapped new towels

A surgeon's preference card indicates the surgeon wears a size L gown and double-gloves with a size 7 inner glove and size 6-1/2 outer glove, and the first assistant wears a size XL gown and double-gloves with a size 7-1/2 inner glove and size 7 outer glove. The first assistant arrives prior to the surgeon. Which of the following is the proper order to place the sterile attire on the back table?

A. L gown, 7 glove, 6-1/2 glove, XL gown, 7-1/2 glove, 7 glove
B. XL gown, 7-1/2 glove, 7 glove, L gown, 7 glove, 6-1/2 glove
C. XL gown, 7 glove, 7-1/2 glove, towel, L gown, 6-1/2 glove, 7 glove
D. L gown, 6-1/2 glove, 7 glove, towel, XL gown, 7 glove, 6-1/2 glove

B. XL gown, 7-1/2 glove, 7 glove, L gown, 7 glove, 6-1/2 glove

Following a surgical procedure, which of the following is the BEST sequence of actions for a surgical technologist to take?

A. Remove sterile drapes, remove gown and gloves, and don a pair of unsterile gloves to aid in the care of the postoperative patient.
B. Remove gown and gloves, don a pair of unsterile gloves to remove drapes from the patient, and remove instruments and supplies from the back table.
C. Remove gown and gloves, don a pair of sterile gloves to remove drapes from patient, and remove gloves and don a pain of unsterile gloves to clean the back table.
D. Remove sterile drapes, remove gown and gloves, and don a pair of sterile gloves to clean back table.

A. Remove sterile drapes, remove gown and gloves, and don a pair of unsterile gloves to aid in the care of the postoperative patient.

Which of the following drugs neutralizes the action of heparin?
A. calcium chloride
B. protamine sulfate
C. lidocaine (Xylocaine)
D. neostigmine (Prostigmin)

B. protamine sulfate

Which of the following wounds is MOST likely in the inflammatory phase of wound healing?

A. a Bankart repair, one week post-procedure
B. a laparotomy incision with a cicatrix
C. an open reduction internal fixation (ORIF) of a finger, two weeks post-procedure
D. an abdominal incision, 20 minutes post-closure

D. an abdominal incision, 20 minutes post-closure

To revascularize the heart muscle of a patient with heart disease, a graft may be anastomosed between which of the following two vessels?
A. internal mammary artery to affected coronary artery
B. subclavian artery to affected coronary artery
C. internal mammary artery to aorta
D. subclavian artery to aorta

A. internal mammary artery to affected coronary artery

A laparotomy drape has been placed on a patient, and unprepped skin on the operative site is exposed. Which of the following is the BEST next step?
A. Apply drapes over unprepped skin.
B. Reposition the drapes closer together.
C. Remove drapes and re-prep.
D. Cover with an adhesive drape.

C. Remove drapes and re-prep

While preparing a sterile field, a surgical technologist secures the Bovie holster to the Mayo stand. The surgeon insists on keeping the Bovie by him toward the head of the patient. Which of the following would be the BEST course of action?

A. Move Bovie holster up by head of patient.
B. Do not move the Bovie holster.
C. Tell the circulator to document the surgeon's response.
D. Remove the Bovie from the field.

A. Move Bovie holster up by head of patient.

Ratcheted instruments should be
A. soaked in a saline solution.
B. prepared for decontamination with curved tips up.
C. opened for washing and sterilizing.
D. sterilized in the sonic washer.

C. opened for washing and sterilizing.

An effective packaging material used for a Balfour to be steam sterilized

A. permits penetration by the sterilant.
B. allows for condensation that produces wet packs.
C. allows for exposure to peracetic acid.
D. is dictated by the surgeon's preference.

A. permits penetration by the sterilant.

The parathyroid gland regulates
A. insulin.
B. calcium.
C. sodium.
D. aldosterone.

B. calcium.

Scoliosis is MOST commonly found in which of the following curves of the vertebral column?

A. cervical

B. thoracic

C. lumbar

D. sacral

B. thoracic

Which of the following is the MOST effective mechanical method of controlling bleeding occurring from needle holes in vessel anastomoses?

A. pledget

B. suction

C. ligature

D. clamp

A. pledget

Which of the following should be visualized on an x-ray to determine if a long bone is still growing?

A. periosteum

B. diaphysis

C. medullary canal

D. epiphyseal plate

D. epiphyseal plate

Which of the following procedures for obtaining an informed consent form is appropriate?

A. The patient is asked to sign the consent form after the surgeon has explained the procedure.

B. The surgical technologist in the circulator role is ultimately responsible for obtaining the signed consent form.

C. The patient is asked to read the entire consent form after signing it.

D. The consent form is witnessed by one member of the patient's family.

A. The patient is asked to sign the consent form after the surgeon has explained the procedure.

Which of the following procedures is used for removal of an embolus?

A. endarterectomy

B. balloon catheterization

C. aneurysmectomy

D. fasciotomy

B. balloon catheterization

Which of the following items should be used to transport a patient in traction?

A. bed

B. stretcher

C. wheelchair

D. fracture table

A. bed

At the conclusion of the surgical procedure, the Mayo stand should

A. remain sterile until the patient leaves the room.

B. be pulled away from the sterile field by the circulator after skin closure.

C. be completely emptied immediately after skin closure.

D. be considered unsterile once the dressing is applied.

A. remain sterile until the patient leaves the room.

Which of the following is used during a tympanoplasty?
A. image intensifier
B. hypothermia unit
C. operating microscope
D. argon laser

C. operating microscope

Removing a cataract by ultrasonic vibration and aspiration is called
A. laser surgery.
B. phacoemulsification.
C. extracapsular extraction.
D. intracapsular extraction.

B. phacoemulsification.

Surgical loupes are used to
A. provide hemostasis.
B. infuse the body cavity.
C. magnify the surgical field.
D. stimulate the circulatory system.

C. magnify the surgical field

A patient undergoing a blood transfusion is having a hemolytic reaction. Which of the following actions should the healthcare providers take FIRST?
A. Administer dantrolene.
B. Stop the transfusion.
C. Monitor urine output.
D. Send blood sample to blood bank.

B. Stop the transfusion

A patient's dentures are removed in the operating room. Which of the following is the proper procedure for the care of the dentures?

A. Return them to the patient's unit and leave them at the nurses' station.
B. Place them in a labeled denture cup and keep them with the patient's chart.
C. Wrap them in a paper towel and give them to the anesthesiologist.
D. Ask the circulator to return them to the patient's room.

B. Place them in a labeled denture cup and keep them with the patient's chart.

Which of the following is associated with secondary intention wound healing?

A. delayed suturing
B. tissue granulation
C. wound dehiscence
D. uncomplicated healing

B. tissue granulation

When inflating a 5-cc balloon on a Foley catheter, which of the following would be the MOST appropriate choice?
A. 3-5 mL of sterile water
B. 3-5 mL of normal saline
C. 8-10 mL of sterile water
D. 8-10 mL of normal saline

C. 8-10 mL of sterile water

During a craniotomy, removal of the bone flap is followed by
A. incision of the dura mater.
B. incision of the galea aponeurotica.
C. application of the Raney clips.
D. suturing of the dura mater.

A. incision of the dura mater

During a laparoscopic appendectomy, which of the following types of staplers should the surgical technologist have ready on the back table for removing the appendix and ensuring no spillage of bowel content?

A. intraluminal
B. linear
C. skin
D. purse-string

B. linear

Which of the following solutions is used to identify diseased areas for a cold conization of the cervix?

A. Lugol's
B. fluorescein
C. methylene blue
D. Isovue

A. Lugol's

Which of the following is the correct position for dilation and curettage?
A. Sims
B. supine
C. Kraske
D. lithotomy

D. lithotomy

An RN has just asked a surgical technologist to complete a task that is within the surgical technologist's scope of practice, but the surgical technologist does not feel comfortable completing the task independently. Which of the following is the surgical technologist's BEST course of action?

A. Ensure that the RN has documented that the task was delegated to the surgical technologist.
B. Request that the RN provides the appropriate level of supervision during the task to ensure safety.
C. Confirm that the initial orientation asked about the surgical technologist's competency for the task.
D. Obtain verbal instructions for completing the task from the RN before she leaves the room.

B. Request that the RN provides the appropriate level of supervision during the task to ensure safety.

Which of the following may be used for a cerebral aneurysm?
A. dura hook
B. nerve hook
C. brain spoon
D. rake retractor

C. brain spoon

Which of the following instruments should be included in the set-up for a laminectomy?
A. Hohmann
B. Mayfield
C. Kerrison
D. Bennett

C. Kerrison

A surgical technologist is preparing a fresh specimen for frozen section to be passed off of the field. How should the specimen be prepared to be passed to the circulator?
A. wrap it in a moist sponge
B. remove any suture material that may be attached

C. wrap it in a Telfa pad

D. remove from back table using a hemostat

C. wrap it in a Telfa pad

Which of the following suturing techniques features short lateral stitches that are taken beneath the epithelial layer of skin?

A. purse-string

B. traction

C. mattress

D. subcuticular

D. subcuticular

Which of the following surgical needles is MOST appropriately used in a liver resection?

A. cutting

B. taper

C. blunt

D. trocar

C. blunt

Which of the following is NOT an acceptable technique when placing a patient in the lithotomy position?

A. arms placed on arm boards

B. legs placed in stirrups one at a time

C. both legs placed in stirrups simultaneously

D. hips placed over the lower break of the table

B. legs placed in stirrups one at a time

What is the function of silver sulfadiazine (Silvadene)?

A. antimicrobial

B. hemostasis
C. irrigation
D. anticoagulant

A. antimicrobial

If unexpected heavy blood loss occurs during an abdominal procedure, a surgical technologist should request additional

A. lap sponges.
B. RAY-TEC sponges.
C. Kitners.
D. cottonoids.

A. lap sponges

A surgical technologist is explaining the steps of the ESU circuit to a student. The surgical technologist should explain that the electric current is channeled back to the generator through the
A. power source.
B. active electrode (ESU pencil).
C. patient.
D. dispersive (inactive) electrode.

D. dispersive (inactive) electrode.

Sponges that have been added to the sterile field after a procedure has begun should be counted by the
A. circulator and surgeon.
B. surgical technologist in the scrub role and surgical first assistant.
C. surgeon and surgical first assistant.
D. surgical technologist in the scrub role and the circulator.

D. surgical technologist in the scrub role and the circulator.

During a procedure, a surgical technologist touches an unsterile item with a sterile glove. Which of the following should be done?

A. Change the glove at once.
B. Break scrub and rescrub.
C. Wait until closing to change the glove.
D. Ask the surgeon what to do.

A. Change the glove at once

The oxygen-carrying capacity of red blood cells is a function of
A. albumin.
B. hemoglobin.
C. hematocrit.
D. prothrombin.

B. hemoglobin.

Which of the following procedures uses a trocar?
A. cystoscopy
B. laparoscopy
C. proctoscopy
D. bronchoscopy

B. laparoscopy

A major function of the colon is to

A. absorb water.
B. secrete hormones.

C. secrete digestive enzymes.

D. absorb the products of digestion.

A. absorb water

Hepatitis B is caused by a
A. prion.
B. virus.
C. protozoan.
D. bacterium.

B. virus.

At the conclusion of a surgical case, how would the surgical technologist in the scrub role aid in reducing bioburden on instruments as the first step in the sterilization cycle?
A. hand cleaning
B. disinfection
C. sorting
D. sterilization

A. hand cleaning

A potential surgical complication of an inguinal herniorrhaphy is injury to the
A. phrenic nerve.
B. sciatic nerve.
C. spermatic cord.
D. femoral artery.

C. spermatic cord.

What type of incision is typically used for an open cholecystectomy?

A. McBurney's

B. Pfannenstiel

C. midline

D. subcostal

D. subcostal

Which of the following pathogens would MOST likely cause a post-operative SSI?

A. Staphylococcus aureus

B. Enterococcus spp.

C. Streptococcus spp.

D. Escherichia coli

A. Staphylococcus aureus

Which of the following must be done before sterilizing an instrument with a lumen?

A. allowing the instrument to dry completely

B. ensuring the stylet is still within the lumen

C. injecting a small amount of distilled water into the lumen

D. wrapping separately in a peel pack pouch and placed in the tray

C. injecting a small amount of distilled water into the lumen

Which of the following is the correct order, from the outermost to the innermost layer, of the tissues that compose the wall of the stomach and small intestine?

1. submucosa

2. muscularis

3. serosa

4. mucosa

A. 1, 4, 2, 3

B. 3, 2, 1, 4
C. 1, 2, 4, 3
D. 3, 4, 2, 1

B. 3, 2, 1, 4

Which of the following is NOT a symptom of shock?
A. tachycardia
B. hypertension
C. cold, clammy skin
D. increased respirations

B. hypertension

When transferring an unconscious, post-operative adult patient from the operating room table to a bed, what is the minimum number of people required for safe transfer?
A. 1
B. 2
C. 3
D. 4

D. 4

Which of the following scissors is MOST likely found in a basic hysterectomy set-up?
A. Potts-Smith
B. Stevens
C. Jorgenson
D. Iris

C. Jorgenson

Which of the following is used to remove clots and tissue from the bladder during transurethral resections (TURPs)?

A. lithotrite
B. asepto syringe
C. Ellik evacuator
D. Fogarty catheter

C. Ellik evacuator

A Javid shunt is used for which of the following procedures?

A. carotid endarterectomy
B. femoral-popliteal bypass
C. abdominal aneurysmectomy
D. saphenous vein ligation

A. carotid endarterectomy

How much 0.25% bupivacaine (Marcaine) should be mixed with 1 mL of 1.0% lidocaine (Xylocaine) to make the solution equal strengths of both medications?

A. 2.0 mL
B. 4.0 mL
C. 5.0 mL
D. 10.0 mL

B. 4.0 mL

Hair removed during preparation for cranial surgery should be

A. discarded by the circulator.
B. sent to pathology.
C. used for potential reimplantation.
D. saved because it is personal property.

B. sent to pathology

Which of the following terms best describes a formal medical process when death occurs in surgery and the surgeon and anesthesia care provider must verify that death has occurred?

A. determination of death
B. rigor mortis
C. postmortem procedures
D. livor mortis

A. determination of death

To help prevent toxicity and vascular events in a patient where polymethylmethacrylate (PMMA) is used, which of the following devices should a surgical technologist have available?
A. pulse lavage
B. mask
C. smoke evacuator
D. cement mixer with charcoal filter

A. pulse lavage

A pneumatic tourniquet may be used for extremity surgery to
A. exsanguinate the extremity.
B. allow the surgeon more operating time.
C. reduce blood loss.
D. create an anesthetic effect.

C. reduce blood loss.

During a craniotomy, which of the following types of bone is entered?

A. flat

B. round

C. long

D. short

A. flat

Which of the following is a procedure for removing excess skin from the face and neck?

A. rhinoplasty

B. rhytidectomy

C. cheiloplasty

D. blepharoplasty

B. rhytidectomy

During an open repair of an indirect hernia, which of the following drains should a surgical technologist have available to pass the surgeon once the spermatic cord has been dissected?

A. Malecot

B. T-tube

C. Jackson-Pratt

D. Penrose

D. Penrose

What color is a nitrous oxide tank?

A. blue

B. gray

C. green

D. orange

A. blue

Which of the following is MOST likely to be in place while transferring a patient from the operating room table to the stretcher?

1. IV tubing
2. Fogarty catheter
3. EKG wires
4. Foley catheter

A. 1 and 2 only
B. 1 and 4 only
C. 2 and 3 only
D. 3 and 4 only

B. 1 and 4 only

Which of the following types of sponges is used directly on the structures of the brain?
A. RAY-TEC
B. cherry
C. Weck-cel
D. cottonoid

D. cottonoid

Which of the following procedures requires an incision in the suprasternal notch?

A. mediastinoscopy
B. bronchoscopy
C. parotidectomy
D. pericardectomy

A. mediastinoscopy

Following an abdominal surgery, the surgeon has just closed the peritoneum. Which of the following layers will be sutured next?

A. fascia

B. muscle

C. subcutaneous

D. subcuticular

A. fascia

During the application of arch bars, the surgeon will MOST likely use which of the following between the teeth and around the bar?

A. 0-1 Dexon

B. 5-0 to 6-0 Vicryl

C. 25- or 26-gauge stainless steel wire

D. 35- or 40-gauge stainless steel wire

C. 25- or 26-gauge stainless steel wire

In which of the following positions should a patient be placed for a low anterior colon resection?

A. dorsal recumbent

B. prone

C. lateral

D. lithotomy

D. lithotomy

A #12 knife blade on a #7 handle is MOST commonly used for what type of surgery?

A. gastrectomy

B. hysterectomy

C. adenoidectomy

D. tonsillectomy

D. tonsillectomy

Which of the following anticoagulants should be given during a vascular procedure to prevent normal blood clotting?

A. heparin sodium
B. protamine sulfate
C. atropine
D. epinephrine

A. heparin sodium

What advantage do hand-held retractors have over self-retaining retractors?
A. less exposure
B. operator dependency
C. lesser fatigue factor
D. dynamic adjustability

D. dynamic adjustability

In which of the following congenital anomalies does the urethra open on the underside of the penis?
A. chordee
B. epispadias
C. phimosis
D. hypospadias

D. hypospadias

Once a surgical technologist dons a gown, the cuffs on the gown are considered unsterile because they are

A. covered by the cuff of the sterile glove.

B. double thickness.

C. absorbant and collect moisture.

D. stretchable and pliable.

C. absorbant and collect moisture.

A physician prescribed 50 milligrams of Demerol. The Demerol is supplied in 100 mg/mL. How many mL of Demerol should be given?

A. 0.5 mL
B. 1.0 mL
C. 1.5 mL
D. 2.0 mL

A. 0.5 mL

A surgeon asks a surgical technologist to place a drop of a mydriatic solution in OD. As a result of this medication, the pupil of the

A. right eye will dilate.
B. left eye will dilate.
C. right eye will constrict.
D. left eye will constrict.

A. right eye will dilate.

A Marshall-Marchetti-Krantz (MMK) requires which of the following skin preparations?
1. abdominal
2. vaginal
3. rectal
4. extremity

A. 1 and 2 only
B. 1 and 3 only
C. 2 and 4 only
D. 3 and 4 only

A. 1 and 2 only

Which of the following conditions is triggered by an injection of succinylcholine (Anectine) and causes an unusually high fever?

A. osteomyelitis
B. sepsis
C. malignant hyperthermia
D. appendicitis

C. malignant hyperthermia

Which of the following statements regarding surgical scrubbing is NOT true?
A. Two accepted methods of surgical scrubbing are the timed method and the counted brush-stroke method.
B. A vigorous 5-minute scrub with a reliable agent may be as effective as a 10-minute scrub done with less mechanical action.
C. Prolonging a scrub beyond the standard scrub length is effective in decreasing microbe counts.
D. When gloves are removed at the end of a surgical procedure, the hands are contaminated and should be immediately washed.

C. Prolonging a scrub beyond the standard scrub length is effective in decreasing microbe counts.

Which of the following spore-forming microorganisms are used as biological monitors for checking steam sterilization effectiveness for a load of instruments in a rigid container?
A. Bacillus stearothermophilus

B. Bacillus atrophaeus

C. Mycobacterium tuberculosis

D. Streptococcus pyogenes

A. Bacillus stearothermophilus

During a laminectomy, disk material is removed with

A. an osteotome.

B. a Kerrison rongeur.

C. a pituitary rongeur.

D. a periosteal elevator.

C. a pituitary rongeur.

Which of the following retractors is used for a C-section?

A. De Lee

B. Hibbs

C. O'Connor-O'Sullivan

D. Auvard

A. De Lee

A surgical technologist is preparing the incision site for the dressing following a TAH. The patient has developed a hematoma at the incision site. The surgeon has left the room. Which of the following actions should the surgical technologist take?

A. Place a pressure dressing.

B. Cover with Dermabond.

C. Steri-Strip the incision.

D. Have the surgeon return.

D. Have the surgeon return.

Which of the following is a type of herniation that occurs with protrusion of the peritoneal sac and its contents (omentum or abdominal viscera)?

A. epigastric

B. umbilical

C. hypogastric

D. femoral

B. umbilical

Heaney clamps are used MOST frequently for which of the following types of surgery?

A. hysterectomy.

B. lobectomy.

C. cystectomy.

D. gastrectomy.

A. hysterectomy

During a C-section, a surgical technologist passes the surgeon a pair of Metzenbaum scissors and Russian forceps. Which of the following anatomical parts is dissected off the uterus and gently retracted prior to uterine incision?

A. ovaries

B. bladder

C. peritoneum

D. broad ligament

B. bladder

Between each surgical procedure, decontamination of walls involves washing

A. areas that have been splashed with blood or debris.

B. all walls with a disinfectant solution.

C. from the floor up to a 5-foot level with a disinfectant solution.

D. from the floor up to a 5-foot level with a viricidal solution.

A. areas that have been splashed with blood or debris.

Which of the following situations would present a problem when preparing instruments for sterilization using a paper-plastic peel pack?
A. The open end of the paper-plastic peel pack has been sealed with tape.
B. The instruments within the paper-plastic peel pack have been held together with tape to avoid shifting.
C. The instruments should be placed in the paper-plastic peel pack with the rings at the end that was sealed by the manufacturer.
D. A felt-tip marker was used to label the plastic on the paper-plastic peel pack prior to sterilization.

B. The instruments within the paper-plastic peel pack have been held together with tape to avoid shifting.

A patient undergoing a procedure while under general anesthesia begins to experience muscle rigidity, followed by tachycardia, metabolic and respiratory acidosis, and cardiac dysrhythmias. Which of the following is the patient experiencing?
A. septic shock
B. malignant hyperthermia
C. cardiopulmonary arrest
D. pulmonary embolism

B. malignant hyperthermia

Anterior and posterior knee stability is influenced by the dynamics of the

A. cruciate ligaments.
B. joint capsule.
C. patellar tendon.
D. collateral ligaments.

A. cruciate ligaments.

When applying a pneumatic tourniquet preoperatively, which of the following items is used to force blood from an extremity?

A. stockinette
B. Coban
C. tourniquet cuff
D. Esmarch bandage

D. Esmarch bandage

After gowning and gloving, a surgeon activates the DuraPrep applicator and proceeds to prep the patient for surgery. Which of the following is the BEST action to take at this time?

A. Assist the surgeon in draping the patient.
B. Regown and reglove the surgeon.
C. Remove drapes and start over.
D. Inform the supervisor.

B. Regown and reglove the surgeon.

After a lung resection is performed, which of the following BEST describes the placement of the collection unit once it is hooked up to the drainage tubing?

A. at the same level as the insertion tube
B. below the level of the insertion tube
C. above the level of the insertion tube
D. at the level of the patient's feet

B. below the level of the insertion tube

Which of the following methods of hospital sterilization does not corrode metal and passes through woven materials like steam?

A. ionizing radiation
B. Steris
C. glutaraldehyde
D. ethylene oxide

D. ethylene oxide

www.ingramcontent.com/pod-product-compliance
Lightning Source LLC
Chambersburg PA
CBHW080008210526
45170CB00015B/1876